Surviving
Your Heart Attack

Surviving
Your Heart Attack

THE DUKE UNIVERSITY
COMPLETE HEART TREATMENT PROGRAM

James V. Warren, M.D.

and Genell J. Subak-Sharpe

DOUBLEDAY & COMPANY, INC.
GARDEN CITY, NEW YORK
1984

Library of Congress Cataloging in Publication Data
Subak-Sharpe, Genell J.
Surviving your heart attack.
Includes index.
1. Cardiacs—Rehabilitation.   2. Exercise therapy.
3. Heart—Diseases—Treatment.   4. Self-care, Health.
I. Warren, James V.   II. Title.   [DNLM: 1. Heart diseases
—Rehabilitation.   WG 166 S941]
RC682.S838   1984   616.1'2   83–25429
ISBN: 0-385-18767-X

In memory of Saul Blatman, M.D.
. . . and James Halford Warren, M.D.

Acknowledgments

Many people are involved in the creation of any book, and this is no exception. We wish to thank DUPAC patients and staff members for the many hours they spent with us, sharing their experience and insight. We hope that their firsthand accounts and advice will benefit our readers, particularly those who are faced with heart disease.

While we cannot list all the many people who have made this book possible, there are those whose special services cannot be overlooked. These include William G. Anlyan, M.D., Duke University Vice-President for Health Affairs; Andrew G. Wallace, M.D., founder of DUPAC; Robert Rosati, M.D., Medical Director; R. Sanders Williams, M.D., Director of Research; and the many other DUPAC staffers: James A. Blumenthal, Ph.D.; Robert Waugh, M.D.; Frederick Cobb, M.D.; Robert Califf, M.D.; Elizabeth Wagner; Interdeep Carath; Carola Ekelund; Thomas Cobb; Helene Mau; Mary K. Rhodes; Lorrie Basnight; Thomas Hill; Lawrence Spann; Miriam Morey; Dorothy Efland; Karen Kale; Laura Boyce; Patricia Houser; Rita Oden; and Sharon Geer. Special thanks are due F. Paul Koisch, Gloria K. Warren, and Gerald Subak-Sharpe, Ph.D., who were all so instrumental in the creation of the manuscript. Special recognition is also due Roy Norguard, Merle Stone, Michael Jennings, John Hanks, Brodus Crabtree, Ruby McCullers, Lucy Fein, Eleanor Kinney, and Geraldine Mitchell—some of the many DUPAC patients who shared their experiences with us. We are grateful to Vicki Chesler, Emily Paulsen, and Beti Mallett for their editorial and manuscript-preparation services. Our two medical illustrators, Andrea Rainier, who prepared the exercise drawings, and George Schwenck, deserve special thanks for their important services. Finally, we wish to thank our editor at Doubleday, Loretta Barrett, for her patience and invaluable help.

Contents

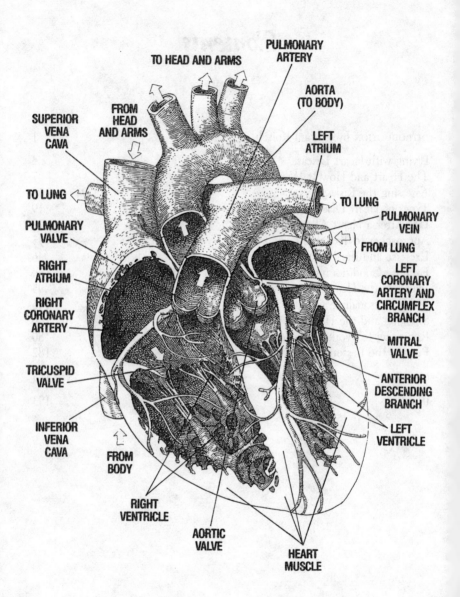

Surviving
Your Heart Attack

Introduction

BY F. PAUL KOISCH

This book is for the millions of American heart patients who are determined to take their future in their own hands but who are uncertain as to how to go about it. No longer is it enough to leave important health decisions to the family physician alone, even though today's doctors have more healing tools at their disposal than at any other time in human history. Good health and its maintenance are an individual responsibility. You can—and should—turn to your doctor for guidance and help, but in the final analysis, you are the one who must make the ultimate decisions and put your doctor's treatment program into practice.

What, then, should the typical heart patient do to control his or her therapeutic outcome? First and foremost, we would urge that heart patients and their families (in short, virtually everyone) learn more about the disease. There is no question that most Americans are uninformed about the nature and treatment of cardiovascular disease. All too often, the knowledge gap is filled with sensational exposés or misinterpreted research data. Providing a basic understanding of the heart and how it works is one of the goals of this book.

This book is also intended to dispel many popular misconceptions about what it means to be a heart patient. To most people, the word "cardiac" implies a person with a sick or damaged heart. In the popular view, a cardiac patient is thought of as someone who is severely limited, slow-moving, sickly; a person whose future is uncertain. This description may apply to some heart patients, but certainly not to the majority. Even patients with severe disease can very often be taught to lead vigorous, productive lives. We have repeatedly demonstrated this at DUPAC (short for the Duke University Preventive Approach to Cardiology), and our findings have been duplicated in many fine cardiac rehabilitation programs elsewhere.

The original concept for DUPAC, as articulated by its founder, Dr. Andrew G. Wallace, was to develop sound approaches to preventing what continues to be our leading health problem. But as the program has evolved,

increasing emphasis has been placed on the cardiac rehabilitation component. Most people who come to DUPAC have had a heart attack or some
other major manifestation of heart disease. They have undergone medical or
surgical treatment and are now seeking guidance on how to get back to the
business of living their lives with a minimum of disability.

Most people who have had a heart attack are filled with disbelief that such
a thing could have happened to them. Very often, the first warning sign of
coronary disease is a heart attack, and in a tragically high percentage of cases
the outcome is sudden death. Fortunately, this picture is changing; an ever-
increasing number of heart-attack patients are surviving the initial event. But
mere survival is not enough; the quality of life is also important.

This book is intended to show you that the quality of life after a heart
attack or other outgrowth of heart disease can, for many people, be even
better than it was before. This may sound like an exaggeration, but I have
seen hundreds of frightened, confused, basically unhealthy people transform
themselves into enthusiastic, optimistic, vigorous individuals in just a few
weeks. How? Through a deceptively simple program of exchanging an unhealthy life-style for one that involves commonsense preventive medicine.
There is nothing radical about DUPAC: it is built around exercise conditioning, dietary modification, stress management, and smoking cessation. While
this may sound too simple to provide the new lease on life that so many
DUPAC participants describe, all of the components are based on careful
research and medical principles.

DUPAC was developed as a clinical program in the Duke Division of
Cardiology. In starting the program, Dr. Wallace, now an Associate Vice-
President of the Duke University Medical Center, developed a new tool for
treating the whole patient, not just the heart, as is so often the tendency in
today's highly specialized practice of cardiology. Dr. Wallace and his colleagues imparted to DUPAC more than sound clinical medicine; they also
brought to the program an esprit de corps and a sense of caring camaraderie
that have contributed to its success. Cardiac rehabilitation may sound like a
deadly serious undertaking; observing a typical DUPAC session quickly dis-
pels any such misconception. There's a sense of fun and even a bit of silliness;
after all, a formerly sedentary, rather portly executive is apt to feel a bit silly
standing on the gym floor in shorts and jogging shoes for the first time in
twenty years.

Heart disease is for life; there are no magic cures or easy treatments that
will make it go away. In this book, the various approaches to treating heart
disease are described. Not all forms of therapy—including exercise—are prescribed for everyone. There are a number of very important considerations
for any heart patient who would like to initiate a DUPAC-style program.
Cardiac rehabilitation has its limits and should not be pursued without medi-

cal guidance. While this book concentrates on DUPAC, widely regarded as a prototype for cardiac rehabilitation, there are many fine programs throughout the United States. You can ask your family physician for referral to one that seems appropriate for you.

Almost any heart patient can benefit from some aspect of rehabilitation. But the long-term effects may take months or years to demonstrate a positive change in cardiovascular health. In most instances, the immediate gains are more likely to stem from the social support and new confidence of testing one's capability and limits in a controlled setting with doctors and emergency equipment close at hand if needed. The fact that they are so seldom needed does not detract from their importance; most people who enroll in a program like DUPAC are afraid to move out on their own. The psychological confidence obtained through regaining one's sense of strength and control surrounded by others is an important factor in any rehabilitation effort.

It would be a grave mistake to assume that the programs and principles outlined in this book are only for heart patients. Research carried out at Duke and other medical centers is providing mounting evidence that heart disease can be prevented through programs of diligent life-style management. The very same therapies used to help heart patients regain function can be employed in a sound preventive program. It is never too early (or late) to start a program of prevention. The children of heart-attack victims should take special note of the urgency to adopt prudent life-style changes. This does not guarantee they will not have a heart attack at some future time, but it does improve the odds against it.

There is one additional benefit that cannot be overlooked, namely a renewed sense of well-being that comes with exercise conditioning, stress management, and other aspects of a healthy life-style. Dr. Wallace has eloquently described this as follows:

> Better health is an important reason why people start to exercise and it is an important dividend. But it's not what keeps people returning [to the exercise field] morning after morning. Rather, it is somehow related to the fact that developing the potential of your body satisfies a basic need, not unlike developing the potential of your brain. Somehow, the ability to contemplate during exercise complements the work of the day and makes it more purposeful and gratifying.

In the final analysis, no one can force better health on another individual. The responsibility is yours alone. For those who choose to consider a healthier life-style as an alternative, this book provides practical and medically sound information.

Mr. Koisch has been Program Director of DUPAC since its founding.

Living with Heart Disease

Although heart disease has been with us since ancient times, it is often referred to as "the twentieth-century epidemic." There are a number of reasons for this. More of us are living to advanced age than ever before in the history of mankind, and the longer we live, the more apt we are to develop heart disease. In many respects, modern life in an urban, industrialized society is bad for the heart. We subject ourselves to excessive stress; millions of us smoke; our typical diet is too high in fat and salt; most of us lead essentially sedentary lives—the list goes on and on. Add to this the fact that we still do not know precisely what causes most forms of heart and blood-vessel disease and you will begin to understand why this remains our number-one health problem.

At least 42 million Americans have one or more forms of heart or blood-vessel disease, which are lumped together under the term "cardiovascular disorders." Millions are unaware that they have a potentially life-threatening illness; they have no obvious symptoms and lead normal lives. Tragically, the first symptom is often sudden death, a heart attack, or a stroke. Others have warnings: chest pain that comes and goes with exertion or emotional upset, high blood pressure that is detected during a routine medical examination, or other symptoms that lead to a diagnosis of cardiovascular disease. A few decades ago, a heart attack or a diagnosis of cardiovascular disease often meant a shortened life marked by increasing disability. Truly remarkable advances since the 1950s have changed this grim prognosis. Today most of the 42 million Americans with cardiovascular disease are able to lead normal, productive lives. More than two out of every three people who suffer a heart attack now survive, and the odds are constantly improving. Even though cardiovascular disease is by far our leading cause of death—claiming more than a million lives a year—the mortality is steadily declining. People with high blood pressure—a disease that afflicts an estimated 37 million Americans—are now able to be treated effectively, thanks to a large number of drugs that have been developed in the past twenty years.

Each year, about 1.5 million Americans suffer heart attacks. A few years ago, about half of them died, often before reaching a hospital. Today more than two thirds survive and most are able to resume normal lives. Advances in treatment—both in and out of the hospital—account for much of the improvement. An array of new drugs, more precise diagnostic techniques, artificial pacemakers and heart valves, and other technological advances take much of the credit. We can now look into the heart itself. Operations such as coronary-artery bypasses and heart-valve replacements, which were unthinkable a few years ago, are now almost routine. In fact, more than 170,000 coronary bypass operations are performed each year, making it one of our most common surgical procedures.

Even though medical science has made many truly marvelous strides forward in the diagnosis and treatment of heart disease, many things are unchanged. Most people are stunned to learn they have cardiovascular disease, even though they may have been repeatedly warned of the risks by their doctors. A heart attack is still an extraordinarily serious and frightening event. Those who survive are haunted by the specter of their own mortality and often emerge from the experience confused and frightened. All too often, they leave the hospital with rather vague instructions like: "Walk a bit each day" or "You better lose some weight" or "Now's the time to stop smoking." All sound advice, but the average person—particularly one who has just had a heart attack—has no idea how to go about following it.

Unfortunately, there are no magic answers or formulas that apply to everyone. Each person must learn how best to live with his or her disease. There are any number of inspiring examples of people who had severe heart attacks and went on to reach new heights—often as a result of their determination to conquer their disease. The late President Lyndon Johnson is one such example. But many others have opted to become cardiac cripples, even when there was no medical need to assume this role. Most fall somewhere in between: they manage to pick up again but are afraid to reach for the heights, all too often because they simply don't know how.

This book is intended to give you the information needed to understand the various forms of cardiovascular disease and to help you regain control over your life. It is based on one of the nation's foremost cardiovascular rehabilitation programs, developed by doctors, researchers, and other health professionals at Duke University Medical Center. The program, known as DUPAC (for the Duke University Preventive Approach to Cardiology), encompasses a total approach to helping heart patients live with their disease. This includes not only the best in medical or surgical treatment but also exercise conditioning; behavior modification; and help in stopping smoking, in diet modification, in coping with stress, and in other aspects of gaining control. There are a number of other fine cardiac rehabilitation programs at medical centers and hospitals throughout the United States, but we have selected DUPAC because of its innovative total approach and pioneering spirit.

In succeeding chapters, the various aspects of DUPAC will be described in detail. Undoubtedly, many of the DUPAC programs can be adapted to your own situation. One important word of caution, however. Before embarking on the exercise regimens, diet, or any other modification in your present life, *check with your doctor.* This is particularly important if you have any form of heart disease. As repeatedly stressed in this book, the intent is to give you knowledge and understanding, not to teach you to be your own doctor. At the same time, it is important to realize that you—and you alone—are responsible for maintaining your own good health. To do this, you should be your doctor's informed partner in your own health care; you should not hesitate to ask your physician about the programs described in this book. There may be good reasons why some are inappropriate for you; chances are, however, your doctor will agree that they make good sense and will tell you how to go about instituting them.

One further word of caution: Although DUPAC researchers have repeatedly demonstrated that most heart patients can benefit from exercise conditioning and other rehabilitation techniques, they are quick to point out the techniques are not a magical cure-all. In the words of Dr. Andrew G. Wallace, founder of DUPAC, "We can't promise any of our patients that they will live one day longer. But we can promise them that they will get more out of living each day!"

The Heart and How It Works

The heart is often likened to a machine—and a marvelously engineered one at that. With truly amazing efficiency, the heart, every minute of every day we live, beats an average of sixty to eighty times, controlling a complex circulatory system that supplies oxygen-rich blood and other nutrients to every cell in the body.

To better understand the kinds of cardiovascular diseases that will be discussed in this book, let us first look at the normal heart and how it works. The heart is a hollow, muscular organ that is divided into two sides: left and right. In turn, each side is divided into two chambers: an atrium, into which blood is collected, and a ventricle, which pumps the blood. The right atrium receives the blood that has circulated through the body. This blood is depleted of oxygen and loaded with carbon dioxide. From the right atrium, it passes to the right ventricle, which pumps it to the lungs via the pulmonary artery. In the lungs, the carbon dioxide is removed from the blood in exchange for a fresh supply of oxygen. The oxygenated blood then returns to the heart, traveling through the pulmonary vein into the left atrium and then to the left ventricle. This chamber is the workhorse pump, responsible for sending the oxygen-rich blood to the circulatory system and, ultimately, to all parts of the body.

The heart is a relatively small organ—about the size of two clenched fists in the average adult—weighing eleven to sixteen ounces. It lies between the lungs in the upper chest cavity. It controls a complex circulatory system made up of a network of arteries that branch into the smaller arterioles. In turn, the arterioles branch into the capillaries, which supply the individual body tissues with oxygen and other nutrients and collect carbon dioxide and other waste products. To return the oxygen-depleted blood to the heart, the capillaries converge into small veins called venules that feed into the larger veins, which carry the blood back to the heart to begin the circulatory cycle anew. An adult man weighing one hundred and fifty pounds has about eleven pints of blood. In a normal, active adult, the heart beats about one hundred thousand times a day, pumping more than four thousand gallons through some sixty thousand miles of blood vessels—a truly prodigious workload that most of us are totally unaware of until something goes awry.

The heart's rhythmic beating action is maintained by a natural pacemaker, a bundle of cells that generate the electrical impulses needed to coordinate the heart's contractions. A system of valves keeps the blood moving in the right direction. Like all body tissues, the heart itself requires a constant supply of oxygen-rich blood. This is supplied by the coronary arteries, so named because they encircle the heart like a crown.

Although the heart rests for only a fraction of a second between beats, it is designed to last a lifetime—conceivably one hundred or more years. Even in the presence of marked disease, the heart can continue to pump enough blood to sustain life, even though activities may be restricted. Until about thirty-five years ago, most people regarded heart disease as either a part of the aging process, the result of rheumatic fever, or part of our genetic makeup; in other words, inevitable events, over which we had little control. But thanks to a number of large-scale studies, most notably the Framingham Heart Study, which began in 1948 and has followed more than five thousand residents of this Boston suburb ever since, we have learned that cardiovascular disorders are not inevitable consequences of aging or heredity. Instead, they are in large part somehow related to the way we live: what we eat, smoke, and drink; how we work and play; how we cope with stress; and how we manage high blood pressure, diabetes, obesity, and other health problems. In short, it has been only in the past few decades that we have come to realize that many heart attacks and strokes can be prevented or delayed by changing our life-styles.

This realization has been paralleled by major advances in the treatment of heart disease. A number of effective drugs have been developed to control high blood pressure. The widespread use of antibiotics has dramatically reduced the incidence of rheumatic heart disease—at one time a leading cause of early cardiac death. Other new drugs are effective in controlling cardiac arrhythmias: disturbances in the heart's natural rhythm. The development of the heart-lung machine in the mid-1950s—a device that can temporarily assume the function of the body's circulatory system—paved the way for open-heart surgery and a number of operations to repair the heart. A few years ago, more than half of all heart-attack victims died before receiving medical help. This figure has probably been reduced in those communities that now have an effective mobile coronary care system with emergency medical teams trained in cardiopulmonary resuscitation, defibrillation, and other lifesaving techniques. Most hospitals now have coronary care units, in which patients are constantly monitored during the crucial few days following a heart attack—an advance that is aimed at reducing the number of in-hospital deaths.

There is growing evidence that this double-headed effort of prevention and improved treatment is paying off. Deaths from cardiovascular diseases have declined in the past decade. But while major gains have been made, the battle has by no means been won. However, even though cardiovascular disease is still our leading health problem, it is something each one of us can do something about. If you are a healthy person under the age of thirty and have no cardiovascular risk factors, then it is probably safe for you to follow the DUPAC program, which is described in the following chapters. Of course, if you are a heart patient, *do not attempt to alter your treatment regimen unless your doctor says you should.* However, if you have any questions or would like to try the DUPAC approach, do not hesitate to ask your doctor; chances are he or she will agree that it can be adapted to your individual needs and will tell you how to go about doing it.

Assessing the Risks

We often hear statements like: "He's at high risk for a heart attack" or "You can lower your risk by doing this or that." But what do we mean when we talk about cardiovascular risk? In this chapter, we will summarize the various circumstances that appear to increase the risk of a heart attack and tell how these various risk factors have been identified. Some are related to our lifestyle (what we eat, whether or not we smoke, how well we cope with stress), and others involve factors over which we have no control (heredity, age, sex).

At the outset, it is important to understand that no one can predict with certainty who is going to have a heart attack. Some people seem to violate all the rules—they smoke, eat all the wrong foods, never exercise, subject themselves to intolerable stress, ignore their doctors' warnings about high blood pressure—and still live to a ripe old age without ever experiencing even a twinge of chest pain. And there are those who seem to do all the right things and still are stricken with a heart attack at an early age. We cannot say why this happens; there are still many unknowns about heart disease. But research is constantly providing new insight and elucidating these unknowns. Although there are exceptions, we know that, in a large enough population group, we can identify a segment whose members will have a higher-than-average incidence of heart attacks by assessing the presence of specific risk factors.

ROLE OF EPIDEMIOLOGY

It has been only in the past few decades that we have identified certain factors that seem to increase the risk of a heart attack. This has been made possible by the study of disease patterns in large population groups—a branch of medicine known as epidemiology. It has long been known that some population groups have a very high incidence of certain diseases, while others seem to be virtually immune. In some instances, the reasons are readily apparent. Snail fever, for example, is a very common parasitic disease in Egypt, Southeast Asia, and certain other tropical countries, but it is virtually unknown in North America and northern Europe. The reason? The snail that harbors the parasite thrives in the Nile and in the rice paddies of Asia but cannot survive in the colder waters of the north. Certain cancers are common in some population groups, geographic areas, or cultures, and very rare in others. Here the reasons are not as apparent as in snail fever, but such things as diet, viral disease, and heredity seem to be important factors. Similarly, heart attacks and coronary heart disease are most common in industrialized countries—the United States, Canada, and northern Europe in particular—and relatively rare in nonindustrialized countries. What is it about our way of life that makes us more vulnerable to heart disease? To arrive at the answer, a number of large-scale epidemiological studies have been conducted over the past thirty years and a number of consistent patterns have emerged from these that have enabled scientists to identify several major cardiovascular risk factors. These are as follows:

Controllable risk factors

- High blood cholesterol
- High blood pressure
- Cigarette smoking
- Sedentary life-style
- Type A personality
- Environmental stress
- Obesity
- Diabetes

Risk factors over which we have no control

- Age (The risk goes up with age.)
- Sex (Men are at higher risk than premenopausal women.)
- Heredity (A family history of heart attack increases the risk.)

ROLE OF DIET

A number of studies have concentrated on eating habits and their relationship to heart disease. One of these studies—the Seven Countries Study, conducted in the 1950s and 1960s—concentrated on dietary patterns. In all, eighteen communities were studied. The highest incidence of heart disease occurred in eastern Finland; followed by Zutphen, in the Netherlands; and among railroad workers in the United States. At the other end of the scale, the lowest incidence was found among men from Corfu and Crete, in Greece; Dalmatia, in Yugoslavia; and Japan. The high death rates seemed to correlate most closely with the consumption of saturated (mostly animal) fats. The eastern Finns consumed 22 percent of their total calories in the form of saturated fats, followed closely by the American railroad workers, with 19 percent. The Finns also had very high levels of blood cholesterol, as did the Americans and the Dutch.

In contrast, the Greeks, who consumed 40 percent of their total calories in the form of fats (comparable to the Finns and the Americans), had a low intake of saturated fat—only 8 percent of the total. The rest of the fat calories came from olive oil and other vegetable oils. The Japanese had one of the lowest intakes of fat—only 9 percent of the total calories, with 3 percent from saturated fats. They also had very low levels of blood cholesterol. But studies performed among Japanese who have moved to Hawaii and California and have adopted a typical high-fat American diet lose their immunity from heart attacks and suffer the same high incidence as their fellow Americans. Other large-scale studies have produced similar results, leading scientists to conclude that a diet high in animal fats and consequently high levels of blood cholesterol constitutes a major cardiovascular risk factor, probably because this leads to a buildup of fatty deposits in the coronary arteries, thus reducing the blood flow to the heart muscle. (The role of high cholesterol in the development of heart disease is discussed in greater detail in the chapter "Diet and the Heart," pages 95–145.)

THE ROLE OF HIGH BLOOD PRESSURE

Many people have the mistaken notion that high blood pressure—or hypertension—has something to do with being "hyper," or under tension. Although stress may play a role in hypertension, and blood pressure rises temporarily during periods of tension or stress, the two are not the same thing. Blood pressure is the amount of force with which the blood is being pumped from the heart through the arteries. Hypertension is the clinical term used to describe a resting blood pressure that is too high for the blood vessels to safely sustain over a long period. The damaging effects of high blood pressure may take years to produce obvious symptoms or consequences such as heart attack or stroke.

Blood pressure is expressed in two numbers, for example 120/80. The higher number is the systolic pressure, meaning it is the maximum force being exerted against the artery walls during the heartbeat. The lower number, the diastolic pressure, is the force exerted while the heart is resting between beats. Although there is still disagreement about what constitutes high blood pressure, most experts now agree that a reading of 140/85 is too high and, at the very least, should be carefully monitored. (See "Types of Heart Disease," pages 22–24.)

High blood pressure is the major cause of strokes—the common term used to describe a serious reduction in the blood flow to the brain. There are several types of strokes; the most common is called cerebral thrombosis and is caused by a blockage of a blood vessel by a clot. Another common form is cerebral hemorrhage, the result of the bursting of a weakened blood vessel. Others may be caused by a ruptured aneurysm, a blood-filled pouch that balloons out from a weakened segment of blood vessel. About 500,000 Americans suffer a stroke each year, resulting in more than 170,000 deaths. Most of these could be prevented by effective control of high blood pressure. In addition, high blood pressure also increases the risk of a heart attack—and the higher the blood pressure, the greater the risk. Epidemiological studies among population groups with a low incidence of high blood pressure—certain Indian tribes in South America and South Pacific islanders, for example—have found a corresponding low incidence of heart disease. Of course, other factors may also be involved. These people tend to eat low-fat diets and have a relative absence of other cardiovascular risk factors as well. In any event, most experts now agree that overall risk of a heart attack can be significantly lowered by identifying people with high blood pressure and bringing it to within normal limits.

THE ROLE OF SMOKING

Cigarette smoking is now considered the major contributing factor in more than 30 percent of all heart attacks. If smoking were to be eliminated, about 225,000 American lives now lost to cardiovascular disease could be saved each year, according to the latest *Surgeon General's Report on Smoking and Health.* In fact, smoking is now thought to kill more people from heart attacks than smoking-related cancers. Men aged forty-five to fifty-four who are heavy smokers are ten times more likely to suffer a heart attack than nonsmokers. Recent studies have shed new light on the effects of tobacco use on the cardiovascular system and indicate that even switching to low-nicotine, low-tar brands does not substantially lower the risk involved. (See "Smoking and the Heart," pages 166–79 .)

THE ROLE OF EXERCISE

Since the turn of the century, Americans have become progressively more sedentary in their work. The automobile, automation of much of our industry, and new forms of passive recreation, such as movies and television, all have combined to lower the amount of physical activity among Americans. Although millions of Americans have, in recent years, sought to remedy this by taking up jogging, tennis, and other forms of exercise, they are but a small segment of the population. The vast majority of Americans are still essentially sedentary; it would be a mistake to think we are a fit population simply because 10 or 12 percent jog.

This overall reduction in physical activity has had several important effects on health. It contributes to obesity and an increase in body fat in relationship to muscle. A lack of exercise leads to a reduction in the body's oxygen transport system. Lack of exercise also lessens our ability to cope with stress.

While it has not been proved that a lack of exercise causes heart disease—or, conversely, that exercise can prevent it—there is a statistical relationship between physical activity and cardiovascular health. A number of studies conducted among people who are physically active in their jobs (dock workers, London bus conductors, mailmen, and others) have found that men in these jobs have a lower incidence of heart attacks when compared to people in more sedentary jobs. More recent studies, of Harvard graduates and British civil servants, found that those who engaged in vigorous leisure activities had a lower incidence of heart attacks, compared to those who were relatively inactive. But the evidence is far from conclusive. The lumbermen and farmers in eastern Finland, for example, lead physically active lives, yet have a very high incidence of heart attacks, attributed largely to their high-fat diets. Such contradictions seem to confirm the conclusion of most experts that a variety of risk factors, rather than a single one, are probably involved in most heart attacks. (See "Exercise and the Heart," pages 46–53.)

THE ROLE OF PERSONALITY TYPE

Most people now recognize that personality and our ability to cope with stress are important in overall health. Recent studies have found that stress and our response to it influence the release of body chemicals that may be instrumental in developing coronary heart disease. Several long-term studies also have correlated personality type with increased risk of heart attack. People with Type A personality—characterized by excessive ambition, aggressiveness, hostility, sensitivity to time urgency, and compulsive behavior—have a significantly higher incidence of heart attacks than the more easygoing, Type B personalities. (See "Stress, Personality, and Heart Disease," pages 146–65.)

THE ROLE OF STRESS

In the past decade, increased attention has been focused on the possible role of stress and our response to it in the development of heart disease. Stress, which can be defined as an imbalance between excessive psychological or physical demands and our ability to cope with those demands, is a normal and expected factor of everyday life. The demands of our jobs, families, friends, living environment, and our own internal emotions all produce stress. Some types of stress are almost overwhelming and difficult for anyone to cope with: the death of a spouse or child, loss of a job, a major illness. There are also those trivial but highly frustrating daily occurrences—waiting in line at the bank or grocery store, missing a train or bus, misplacing an important paper, facing short deadlines—that can be highly stressful to some people and barely noticed by others. In fact, some people seem to thrive on stressful challenges, while others become nervous wrecks. We are all different, and respond to similar situations differently. But there is increasing evidence that people who are under constant stress or who respond poorly to normal, everyday stress have an increased incidence of heart attacks.

In general, stress produces both a psychological response and a physiological one. The psychological response is usually characterized by feelings of apprehension, tension, or nervousness. At the same time, there is likely to be heightened activity of the autonomic nervous system: the heart beats faster, breathing increases, blood pressure rises, muscles tense, and there may be increased sweating. These responses are generally referred to as the "fight-or-flight" reaction—a response that can be lifesaving in a dangerous situation. Handled well, stress can actually improve our performance, but when handled poorly, stress can hinder our ability to cope or perform. Signs that we are not coping well include irritation, feelings of pessimism, fatigue, weakness, inability to sleep, loss of appetite or overeating, headaches, an inability to concentrate or perform at usual levels.

How our response to stress may increase our susceptibility to heart attacks and other illnesses is not known. Recent research, however, has found that people who over-respond to stress also release excessive amounts of adrenal hormones and undergo other physical changes that may set in motion some of the factors that lead to heart disease. Since a certain degree of stress is unavoidable, the best approach to coping with it is to learn effective stress-management techniques. These may include relaxation training and learning new ways of thinking about yourself and your situation. (See "Stress, Personality, and Heart Disease," page 152.)

THE ROLE OF OBESITY

People who are obese, defined as being 20 percent or more above ideal weight for age, sex, and body frame, have a shorter life expectancy than people who are of ideal weight. Life insurance studies have found that the risk of premature death from all causes, including heart disease, is greatest in people who are 30 percent or more above normal weight. A recent report from the Framingham Heart Study declared that obesity should be considered among the major controllable cardiovascular risk factors. Previously, most experts had thought that obesity contributed to other cardiovascular risk factors, such as diabetes, atherosclerosis, high blood pressure, and elevated cholesterol and uric acid, but was not itself a risk factor. This view is now changing, as studies confirm that being substantially overweight increases the risk of heart disease, even in the absence of other risk factors. (See "Diet and the Heart," page 101.)

THE ROLE OF DIABETES

Diabetics have an increased risk of heart attacks and artery disease. Diabetes is characterized by an inability to metabolize carbohydrates, either because of an insufficiency of the hormone insulin or the inability of the body to effectively use the insulin it produces. This results in excessive glucose (a sugar) in the blood, some of which may be excreted in the urine. Poorly controlled diabetes is marked by abnormal swings in blood sugar from very high to very low. This is thought to be a factor in the high incidence of hardening of the arteries (arteriosclerosis) and a buildup of fatty plaque (atherosclerosis) along the artery walls, seen in diabetics. Diabetics also tend to have high levels of cholesterol and triglycerides. Weight control, diet, exercise, and insulin, if needed, all are important elements in keeping diabetes under control and minimizing the added risk of heart disease.

RISK FACTORS OVER WHICH
YOU HAVE NO CONTROL

There are several factors that increase the risk of a heart attack and are beyond our control: age, sex, and heredity. As might be expected, the risk of having a heart attack increases as we grow older, approximately doubling each decade after the age of thirty. Blood pressure also rises as we grow older, perhaps adding to the risk. Even so, it does not seem that old age, in itself, is an inevitable cause of heart disease. There are a number of societies in which people live to remarkably old ages without any evidence of severe heart disease. In fact, although a rise in blood pressure with age is considered normal in this country, there are some societies in which blood pressure remains constant despite advanced age. It would seem, then, that the increased risk that comes with age is actually from the accumulation and worsening of other risk factors and not from the advancing years themselves.

It is well known that men, particularly middle-aged men, have a much higher incidence of heart attacks than women. The reasons for this are unknown, although it does not seem to be a lifelong phenomenon. After the age of sixty, women seem to "catch up" and have about the same incidence of heart attacks as men of the same age. Considerable speculation has centered on the role that female hormones may play in protecting against heart disease. For example, women who have their ovaries removed or undergo an early menopause seem to be prone to heart disease at an earlier age than women who undergo menopause in their late forties or early fifties. But men who have been given female hormones do not have a lowered incidence of heart disease; in fact, the opposite occurs. Also, women who take oral contraceptives that contain estrogen have an increased risk of heart attacks and strokes. This is particularly true of women who smoke while using oral contraceptives.

A number of other factors may explain why women enjoy a lower risk of heart disease. They tend to have higher levels of high-density-lipoprotein (HDL) cholesterol, which is considered protective against coronary disease, than men and, until recently, did not smoke in as great number or as heavily as men. It should be noted, however, that there has been an increase in the number of heart attacks among women in their thirties and forties in recent years. While women in this age group still lag far behind men in the total number of heart attacks, the trend is pronounced enough to prompt many experts to speculate that women may be "catching up" with men in this area.

A number of possible explanations are cited, including the increase in smoking among women and the added stress of competing in the job market.

Family history has long been recognized as an important risk factor and one over which we obviously have no control. If your parents, uncles, brothers, sisters, or other close family members suffered heart attacks at an early age, your chances of following suit are greatly increased. A number of risk factors, such as high blood pressure and a hereditary type of elevated cholesterol called familial hypercholesterolemia, run in families and may, in part, explain the increased risk. If there is a family history of early heart disease, especially before the age of fifty or fifty-five, it is particularly important to undergo regular medical checkups and to control or avoid as many of the lifestyle risk factors as possible to minimize your chances of an early heart attack.

SUMMING UP

While we cannot predict who will and who will not have a heart attack on the basis of risk factors alone, it makes sense to reduce or control as many of them as possible. By keeping cholesterol and blood pressure under control, not smoking, maintaining ideal weight, learning how to cope with stress and modifying Type A behavior, and engaging in regular physical activity, we can greatly improve our chances of avoiding a heart attack.

Types of Heart Disease

There are dozens of disorders affecting the heart and blood vessels, and although more than 42 million Americans have some form of cardiovascular disease, the vast majority are able to live relatively normal, productive lives. Treatments vary widely and may include the use of drugs, surgery, diet, and exercise. But no matter what the problem or therapy, the most important member of the treatment team is you, the patient. And the more you know about your heart and how to take care of it, the better. This does not mean you can be your own doctor, but it does mean you can be your doctor's informed partner. In this chapter, we will review the major forms of cardio-vascular disease and what is known about their causes.

CORONARY HEART DISEASE

Also known as coronary artery disease and coronary atherosclerosis, this disorder involves the progressive narrowing, or "hardening," of the blood vessels that nourish the heart muscle. Coronary heart disease almost always entails the buildup of fatty deposits along the artery walls. These deposits, known as fatty plaque, or atheroma, are made up of cholesterol and other fats, and fibrous tissue such as collagen.

We do not know what causes coronary atherosclerosis. It appears to be a lifelong process, beginning in our early years. It is seen most often in popula-tion groups whose diet is high in cholesterol and saturated fats; for example, a diet high in red meats, butter, milk, cheese, and eggs—the sort of fare fa-vored by many Americans. High blood pressure and diabetes appear to exac-erbate the process, and people with these disorders have an increased risk of heart attacks.

There are a number of theories about what might trigger coronary atherosclerosis. The most common theory is that something injures the smooth tissue (endothelium) lining the artery walls. The nature of the initial injury is unknown; some researchers speculate that it may result from biochemical changes prompted by chronic stress or emotional turmoil, such as might be expected in people with Type A behavior. Others think it might be an autoimmune reaction, and still others speculate it is related to changes in blood pressure. Once injured, the arterial wall becomes more susceptible to the buildup of fatty deposits. These deposits cause further reaction within the artery wall, resulting in the buildup of fibrous, scarlike tissue in addition to the fatty accumulation.

It may take many years for the disease to progress to the point where symptoms occur. A coronary artery can be more than half blocked before there is any serious reduction in blood flow. But as the vessels become increasingly clogged, the amount of blood available to the heart is diminished. About 5 percent of the total amount of blood pumped by the heart each minute goes through the coronary arteries. Since heart muscle is the body's most efficient when it comes to extracting oxygen from the blood, this amount of blood flow ordinarily is enough to meet the heart's demands. But any increased demand on the heart (running to catch a bus, a rise in blood pressure, an emotional upset) increases its need for oxygen. If the coronary arteries cannot deliver this needed blood, symptoms such as shortness of breath and chest pain may occur.

Sometimes the artery may become completely blocked by a clot (coronary thrombus) or by a portion of the fatty plaque that may break away from the artery wall and then become lodged in a narrowed vessel. When this happens, the portion of heart muscle that is normally nourished by that vessel is deprived of oxygen and dies, leading to a heart attack. The medical term for this is myocardial infarction, which means heart-muscle death. Most heart attacks seen in this country are the result of coronary atherosclerosis. Thus, preventing or delaying the buildup of fatty deposits in the coronary arteries is a major objective of any preventive cardiology program.

Most people with coronary heart disease are unaware of the problem until it reaches an advanced stage. Indeed, in a tragic number of cases the first symptom is a heart attack, or sudden cardiac death. Although there is no simple screening test, such as we have for high blood pressure, there are a number of diagnostic tools for determining the extent of coronary disease. An abnormal exercise-tolerance test, for example, may indicate the presence of coronary disease (although it should be noted that this test is not definitive). Very high levels of cholesterol and triglycerides in the blood are common precursors of coronary atherosclerosis, and anyone with high blood lipids should be doubly aware of other possible symptoms. If serious coronary heart disease is suspected, your doctor may want you to undergo coronary angiography (special X-ray studies of the heart and the coronary arteries) or other tests designed to assess heart function.

Chest pain is the most common symptom of coronary heart disease. This pain, known as angina pectoris, is caused by a reduction in oxygen to the heart muscle. Angina usually lasts only a few minutes; it is most often provoked by exercise, emotional unrest, exposure to the cold, or other situations that increase the heart's work load. Rest and the use of nitroglycerin—or some other drug that increases the blood flow to the oxygen-starved (ischemic) heart muscle—will in most instances bring the episode to an end. Typically, anginal pain is described as a pressing or squeezing sensation that begins in the center of the chest. It may spread to the shoulders or the arms (most often along the left side although the right also may be involved), the back, the neck, or the jaw. Although the pain usually goes away within minutes, and most people with angina learn to adjust their pace accordingly, it is vital to heed this important warning sign. Early diagnosis of coronary heart disease and appropriate treatment can reduce or eliminate the episodes and may prevent a heart attack.

There are some cases in which the angina occurs while sleeping or at rest. This pain may be caused by a spasm in a coronary artery. The spasm usually occurs in a diseased artery, but it is also seen in healthy vessels. Again, early diagnosis is important, since coronary spasm usually can be prevented by drug therapy.

The pain of a heart attack is almost always more severe and lasts longer than an attack of angina. Many people experience warning symptoms in the form of vague chest pains or an increase in anginal attacks, often without any obvious cause. Others may suffer a heart attack without any previous warning or precipitating cause. The pain of a heart attack usually does not go away, the way angina does. Untreated, it may last for hours and vary in intensity from mild discomfort to excruciating pain. Sweating, nausea and vomiting, dizziness or fainting, and a feeling of impending doom also may be present. But there are exceptions: 10 percent or more of heart-attack patients do not experience severe pain, and some are unaware that they have had an infarction until it is detected at some later date on an electrocardiogram.

A heart attack is always a medical emergency. If you suspect a heart attack, seek medical help immediately. If an emergency medical squad is available, it should be summoned first. If not, get someone to drive you to the nearest emergency room or hospital with a coronary-care unit; don't try to drive yourself. Many people delay seeking medical help, thinking the pain will pass. Others try to reach their doctors before calling the emergency squad; it's much better to call the emergency service first and then alert your doctor to meet you at the emergency room or hospital.

Of course, not all chest pain originates with the heart. It can come from the lungs, esophagus, or even abdominal organs, such as the stomach. In fact, many people suffering a heart attack initially think they have a gastric problem, such as heartburn or indigestion. Similarly, many suspected heart attacks turn out to be of some other origin. Other causes of chest pain include emotional stress, inflammation of the chest muscles, and diseases of the spine or bony structure of the chest. Pain of muscular or skeletal origin usually can be easily distinguished from heart pain, because it is clearly related to movement or taking a deep breath. Pain triggered by stress or anxiety generally stays in one place, often in the mid-chest, and is accompanied by fast breathing (hyperventilation), a rapid heartbeat, fatigue, and fear. In any event, it is better to err on the side of caution and seek prompt medical attention for an unusual bout of chest pain.

HIGH BLOOD PRESSURE

About 37 million Americans have high blood pressure, or hypertension. This means that the blood moves through the arteries at a greater than normal force or pressure. A number of factors influence blood pressure, beginning with the heartbeat itself. Each time the heart contracts, about three ounces (one hundred milliliters) of blood is forced into the aorta, the large artery leading from the heart. This creates a sudden surge reflected in the pulse you can feel by pressing on an artery in your wrist, behind your ear, or at some other pulse point. The pressure within the arteries during this phase, when the heart is contracting, is called the systolic pressure and is the higher of the two numbers in a blood-pressure reading (for example, 120/80). The pressure falls when the heart is resting momentarily between beats, and at its lowest point it is called the diastolic pressure. This pressure is determined by the resistance to the flow of blood from the arterioles (the smallest arteries) into the capillaries. If for some reason these arterioles are narrowed or constricted, there will be greater resistance and the diastolic pressure will rise. This, in turn, forces the systolic pressure up in order to keep the blood flowing.

Blood pressure can be measured directly by inserting a pressure-sensitive device into an artery. This gives the most accurate reading, but it is generally reserved to a hospital setting; for example during surgery, when a permanent record of blood pressure may be desired. The easier, more familiar method involves using an instrument called a sphygmomanometer, which is taken from the Greek words *sphygmos*, meaning pulse, and *metron*, measure. It has an inflatable cuff that wraps around the arm, a rubber bulb to inflate the cuff, and a device to measure the pressure, which is given in millimeters of mercury. When the cuff is inflated, it momentarily cuts off the flow of blood. The air is then released, and blood begins to flow through the artery. By listening for characteristic sounds through a stethoscope placed on the artery just below the cuff and noting the height of the column of mercury, the highest (systolic) and lowest (diastolic) pressures can be measured. In recent years, a number of simpler, digital blood-pressure devices have been developed that are intended for home use. Most of these devices have a cuff and a digital readout; a stethoscope is not needed. Many of these are not quite as accurate as the devices used by doctors but may be useful for home monitoring by patients with unstable blood pressure or for people who want the reassurance that their treatment is working and their blood pressure is under control. In any instance, patients who plan to monitor their blood pressure at home should be instructed by their physicians first.

In about 90 percent of all cases, the cause of hypertension is unknown. In the remaining 10 percent, the causes range from kidney abnormalities, tumors of the adrenal glands, or a congenital defect of the aorta. In these latter cases, the high blood pressure can usually be corrected by treating the underlying cause. No matter what the cause, controlling the high blood pressure is very important if one is to avoid the long-term consequences of the disease, which can be life-threatening. For example, persistent high blood pressure weakens the blood vessels, greatly increasing the risk of stroke. Although the incidence of stroke has fallen markedly in recent years, largely because of the improved detection and treatment of high blood pressure, the five hundred thousand new strokes each year still represent a major public-health problem.

Untreated high blood pressure is also a major risk factor for heart attacks and also can cause an enlargement of the heart, which may eventually lead to congestive heart failure. High blood pressure is very hard on the kidneys; kidney failure is a common outcome of untreated hypertension. The eyes are still another organ vulnerable to persistent high blood pressure; permanent eye damage or even blindness can result from untreated hypertension.

Who gets high blood pressure? As noted, in most cases the cause of hypertension is unknown, but certain factors seem to increase the risk. For example, the disease tends to run in families; if your parents and other close relatives have high blood pressure, your risk of developing it may be higher than normal. Children born to hypertensive parents tend to have blood pressure that is in the high normal range from a very early age on. Many doctors recommend that these high normals be monitored and preventive measures such as a low-salt diet and weight control be started at an early age. Blacks tend to have more hypertension than whites, for reasons that are unknown. Obesity is a major risk factor in developing hypertension, and in many overweight hypertensives, losing weight will return the blood pressure to normal. A high salt intake is often implicated in high blood pressure. While certain types of hypertension respond to a low-salt diet, it has not been conclusively proved that salt causes high blood pressure. Since high blood pressure is rare in societies that have a low-salt diet—desert nomads, for example—researchers have theorized that our high salt intake may account for the high incidence of hypertension. Further study is needed to prove this; in the meantime, reducing salt intake among those who may be susceptible to the disease certainly can do no harm and may be an effective means of prevention.

Other factors that can affect blood pressure include age: as we grow older, our blood vessels lose some of their elasticity and our blood pressure goes up to compensate for this. Certain drugs, such as oral contraceptives, also may increase blood pressure. Many people associate stress with high blood pressure; while tension and emotional unrest can temporarily increase blood pressure, it has not been proved that this is a cause of sustained hypertension.

A blood-pressure reading of 120/80 is considered ideal. Of the 37 million Americans with hypertension, about 20 million are classified as mild, meaning the diastolic pressure ranges from 85 to 104 millimeters of mercury. A few years ago, patients with mild hypertension were monitored every six months or a year, and if the diastolic pressure rose above 105 or so, drug treatment would be initiated. More recently, however, a number of studies have shown the benefits of treating even mild hypertension that persists for more than six months and remains elevated despite more conservative measures, such as reducing salt intake, losing excess weight, and exercising. There is still some debate in the medical community over the point at which drugs should be given to treat mild hypertension. There is no debate, however, over the treatment of moderate to high blood pressure; the benefits in lowered risk of stroke, heart attacks, kidney failure, and other complications are well documented. In addition, a host of highly effective new antihypertensive drugs have been introduced in recent years, making it possible for doctors to adjust dosages and combinations of drugs to come up with an effective regimen that carries the minimum of side effects.

IRREGULAR HEARTBEATS

Any disturbance in the regularity of the heart's beat is referred to as cardiac dysrhythmia, or arrhythmia. The heart has its own electrical system, which stimulates it to beat in a regular, rhythmic fashion. The core of this system is called the sinus node; it is situated in an area on the upper right side of the heart. It generates the electrical impulses that are transmitted to specialized fibers and cells that regulate the contractions of the two pumping chambers. These impulses can be picked up by electrodes placed at certain locations on the chest wall and limbs and recorded on an electrocardiogram —a tracing that shows the electrical activity of the various parts of the heart.

The heart can speed up or slow down according to the demands placed on it. From time to time, everyone experiences a skipped beat, or periods when the heart seems to race. These irregularities generally are only momentary and not a cause for concern. However, there are instances in which the heart's rhythm goes awry and can produce life-threatening disruptions in the heart's function. The beat may be too fast (tachycardia) or too slow (brady-cardia) or marked by abnormal beats, such as premature ventricular contractions, in which the pumping chamber contracts before the next regular beat.

A number of factors can disturb normal heart rhythm; excessive use of caffeine, cigarette smoking, anxiety, and certain drugs are common examples. Congenital heart defects, coronary disease, an overactive thyroid, and some lung disorders also can upset normal heart rhythm. Sometimes otherwise healthy people will experience a fluttering sensation in the chest accompanied by a feeling of fullness, shortness of breath, and light-headedness. This may be a single episode of what is called atrial fibrillation or become a recurrent problem. Such episodes should be investigated; in the case of recurring rhythm disturbances, drugs may be prescribed to control the irregularities.

Although most cardiac arrhythmias are temporary and not a cause for worry, there are some that are life-threatening. One of the most serious is ventricular tachycardia, a condition in which there are more than two consecutive premature beats at a heart rate of more than one hundred beats per minute. This type of arrhythmia can quickly degenerate into a disorganized beating called ventricular fibrillation, in which the heart fails to pump blood. If normal rhythm is not restored, death will result.

In some people, normal heart rhythm cannot be maintained with drugs, and an artificial pacemaker is needed. These devices are generally implanted under the skin with electrodes leading to the heart. The pacemaker supplies the electrical impulses that stimulate the heart to beat in a regular manner. There are two basic types of artificial pacemaker: demand (synchronous) models, which take over whenever the patient's heart rate falls below a predetermined level, and fixed-rate (asynchronous), which deliver constant impulses at a predetermined rate.

CONGESTIVE HEART FAILURE

Heart failure occurs when not enough blood is pumped to meet the body's need for oxygen and nutrients during rest and normal activities. When this happens, the volume of blood builds up, causing an accumulation of fluids, or congestion. Early symptoms of heart failure include a swelling of the legs and difficulty breathing, especially when lying down, which causes the fluid to accumulate in the lungs.

Congestive failure may be caused by damage to the heart muscle, either from a heart attack or a disease of the muscle itself—a condition called cardiomyopathy. Diseases of the heart valves, which prevent adequate flow of blood into the pumping chambers, may also cause congestive failure. Chronic hypertension is still another common cause of congestive heart failure.

Prevention is the best treatment for congestive failure. Anyone who has high blood pressure or valvular disease should be treated to forestall heart failure. Early diagnosis and treatment, either with drugs or surgery or a combination of the two, are important to prevent the heart from deteriorating to the point where it can no longer pump enough blood to meet the body's needs.

HEART-VALVE DISEASE

The flow of blood through the heart's chambers and then into the major vessels that carry it to other parts of the body is controlled by a series of valves. Blood returning to the heart through the venous system passes from the right atrium through the tricuspid valve into the right ventricle. It then travels through the pulmonary valve into the pulmonary artery and the lungs, where it exchanges carbon dioxide for a fresh supply of oxygen. The blood returns to the left atrium and then through the mitral valve into the left ventricle. From this pumping chamber, it is propelled through the aortic valve into the aorta and the circulatory system.

All the valves are made up of thin leaflets of tissue, which, when closed, prevent a backflow of blood, and when open, enable the blood to move to its next destination. A defective valve is one that fails to either open or close properly. When a valve fails to close, for example, there is a backflow (regurgitation) of blood into the chamber from which it has just flowed. This means that there will be even more blood that has to be pumped at the next heartbeat, and eventually the extra work may cause damage to the heart muscle. A valve that fails to open properly (stenosis) also puts an extra strain on the heart; it also may result in an inadequate blood supply to the rest of the body. Abnormal heart rhythms, shortness of breath, and swelling (edema) are common symptoms of advanced heart valve disease.

There are a number of ways in which the heart valves can be damaged, the most common being an infection such as rheumatic fever or a congenital defect. Often people can live with a defective heart valve for years without being aware of the condition. For example, a condition called mitral valve prolapse is very common; it may be present in up to 7 percent of the population. In most people, it is not a serious disorder and causes few if any symptoms. In others, it may produce irregular heartbeats, chest pain, and other symptoms that may be alarming but usually are not serious. The defective heart valve, however, is more susceptible to infection; a severe disease called bacterial endocarditis can follow surgery or even a minor dental procedure. Any symptoms that suggest heart valve disease should be investigated, so that treatment can be undertaken before there is extensive heart damage. In some cases this will mean avoiding infection by taking antibiotics; in others, it may entail taking digitalis or some other drug to slow the heartbeat and increase the heart's efficiency. Diuretics and a low-salt diet may be prescribed to prevent a buildup of fluids.

When the valves are severely damaged, surgery may be recommended to replace them. In recent years, a number of highly efficient artificial valves have been developed, making valve-replacement surgery a relatively common operation.

SUMMING UP

There are a number of other heart and blood-vessel disorders, but these are the main causes of cardiac problems afflicting Americans. Most are highly treatable, and with early diagnosis and appropriate preventive action, they need not advance to disabling or life-threatening stages. As emphasized earlier, millions of Americans are living full, productive lives despite having some form of heart disease. The DUPAC program, described in the following chapters, is specifically designed to achieve this goal.

Life After a Heart Attack

At first glance, it would seem that it's a diverse group of men and women who have gathered in the DUPAC conference room. They represent all ages and economic and educational levels, but they have one very important factor in common: all have had at least one heart attack or have undergone coronary bypass surgery. And all readily admit that this has markedly changed their lives.

Gerald S., a New York City professor, was fifty-six when he had his heart attack. He was walking home carrying a bag of groceries when his legs suddenly felt unbearably weak. He set the bag down to rest for a moment, and the next thing he knew, he was lying on the sidewalk, looking up dazedly at his worried wife, two policemen who had been nearby, and a group of bystanders. He felt weak, but there was no pain. He had had a similar fainting episode at his college the day before, but after a night's rest, he had felt well enough to teach his classes and carry on as usual. He had not seen his doctor after the earlier fainting but had talked to him on the phone. This time, however, an ambulance was called and he was taken to a nearby emergency room. Tests showed that although he did not experience chest pains typical of a heart attack, he had indeed suffered one. Enzyme and other studies indicated it had been a mild heart attack, limited to a small area of the right ventricle, rather than the more vital, left-side, pumping chamber.

Over the next week, he seemed to make a good recovery: he walked for a few minutes every hour or so and, although he was anxious and worried, his progress was uneventful. All in all, he had been a high-risk candidate for a heart attack. Over the previous few years, he had put on about thirty extra pounds. He had high blood pressure but had not been terribly diligent about taking his medication or having the pressure checked regularly. With the stress of his job and family obligations, he had become increasingly inactive physically—there never seemed to be time for a long walk, swimming, or tennis, all activities that he had enjoyed in the past. Now that he had had a heart attack, he knew he would have to change his life-style, even though he was unsure as to how to go about it.

Just before he was to be discharged, his doctor decided he should undergo a very moderate exercise test, just to make sure that his heart was strong enough to cope with normal activities at home. As it turns out, this test probably saved his life: it revealed serious abnormalities; and subsequent coronary angiography showed he had two severely blocked coronary arteries. Instead of going home, as he had planned, he remained in the hospital and underwent coronary-artery bypass surgery.

John H., a music teacher in his early forties, seemed in the peak of health. He played a hard game of tennis, swam almost daily, and was unaware of any cardiovascular risk factors. Then, one day, he suddenly suffered severe chest pains while playing tennis. They passed in a few minutes, but he took the episode as a warning to see his doctor. A complete checkup found he had high blood cholesterol and showed an abnormal exercise test. His doctor advised further tests, including coronary angiography, which confirmed serious coronary disease. He, too, underwent bypass surgery, but, unlike Gerald, he emerged from the operation feeling much weaker than before. "I couldn't walk up even one flight of stairs," he recalled, "and I was on five different drugs."

Brad C., a fireman in his early thirties, was on vacation in Colorado when stricken with a heart attack, followed by a second one two weeks later. His mother had suffered a heart attack when she was only thirty-two, but he had always assumed he was somehow immune. Physically strong and lean, he looked the picture of health, and his job demanded physical fitness. But he had an extremely high cholesterol level, indicating an inherited disease called familial hypercholesterolemia, in which the body manufactures excessive cholesterol, especially when the diet is high in saturated fats. People with this disorder often have heart attacks at very early ages unless steps are taken to decrease the cholesterol. Brad made a satisfactory recovery from his second heart attack but was warned that he must drastically change his diet and that he also must give up his job. "I grew up on ham, fried foods, whole milk— everything I shouldn't eat," he explained. "Changing my diet was hard, but I felt I had no choice. Giving up my job as a fireman was even harder. The Police Department offered me a desk job, but it just isn't the same. . . ."

Geraldine M., a retired social worker, had always been active—she'd walked daily, done a lot of volunteer work, spent time with her family and friends. She had considered herself basically healthy until suffering two heart attacks in less than a year. "I thought I was doing all the right things," she recalled, "and I was set for a healthy, active retirement. But after my second heart attack, I could barely walk and I was terribly depressed."

As they talked about their experiences, all remembered the fears and doubts that seemed to dominate their lives after their heart attacks or bypass operations. "I was afraid to walk across the room," Brad, the ex-fireman said. "I didn't know how much I could do, or even who to ask. My doctor told me to try walking a few blocks at a time, but I didn't know how fast I should go, or whether I should climb hills or stairs." Gerald had similar doubts: "I would feel my heart pounding, and I would think I might be having another heart attack." Geraldine described the fear as paralyzing: "I would feel a twinge, and be terrified that this was another heart attack." Their experiences are not unusual; if you or someone close to you has had a heart attack or serious coronary disease, you undoubtedly will recognize the feelings of the patients quoted here. Virtually everyone who has a heart attack emerges from the experience full of fear. Anxiety and depression are common. Many are angry and frustrated; others feel dejected and resigned to a life filled with restrictions and disability. Most recover determined to change—lose weight, stop smoking, exercise regularly—but are confused as to how to achieve these goals.

"Our first task," says DUPAC founder Dr. Andrew G. Wallace, "is to determine just how much patients can do, and then to get them on their feet and feeling better. Once they realize that they aren't going to keel over walking around the track a few times, they begin to regain their confidence and optimism. And we have found that even severely damaged hearts can still function well enough to permit a reasonably normal life. The important thing we try to teach is to focus on those things you can still do, rather than concentrate on the negatives."

Two thirds of the nearly 1.5 million Americans who have heart attacks each year now survive, a marked improvement from the 50 percent mortality of a decade ago. Just as important, most survivors are capable of leading relatively normal lives. Most can return to their jobs, resume their sex lives, travel, engage in favorite recreational pursuits. Of course, some adjustments may be necessary. A heart attack, by definition, leaves permanent damage. In some, this may be relatively minor; in others, the damage may be severe enough to impose certain limitations. Like Brad, for example, some heart-attack patients will need to seek less strenuous jobs. Others may need physical rehabilitation to regain the use of certain weakened muscle groups. Unfortunately, there is still a tendency on the part of many physicians and heart patients alike to elect disability, rather than rehabilitation. Heart disease remains the leading cause of disability among Americans under the age of sixty-five. According to the American Heart Association, more than a half million Americans are receiving disability benefits because of cardiovascular diseases, at an annual cost of $12.4 billion. The DUPAC program, which includes occupational rehabilitation in its total approach, has demonstrated that a large percentage of those heart patients who would ordinarily elect early retirement can instead return to their jobs or seek other employment.

"Staying active has been the single most important factor in my recovery," says Merle S., a longtime Duke participant. "After I had my heart attack, all I thought about were the things I couldn't do: I couldn't eat salty or fatty foods; I couldn't drive alone; I couldn't work as hard. DUPAC taught me that I still could eat the things I really like; I could walk five miles and feel great; I not only could drive, I could also ride a bicycle; and I could return to my job with a healthier outlook than I had before. In short, I learned to live every day to the fullest, and stop worrying about tomorrow."

In discussing their common concerns and problems, this group of DUPAC patients agreed that the two most important elements in successful rehabilitation are knowledge and being able to discuss their concerns not only with their doctors but also with people who have had the same problem.

"I didn't even understand what was meant by a heart attack," Gerald, the New York professor, confessed. "I had a vague idea that it involved some sort of blockage in the heart, but beyond that I was totally ignorant." Learning how the heart functions and what had happened in his specific heart attack and subsequent bypass surgery helped him understand that the damage had been slight and that the potential for another heart attack had been greatly diminished by the coronary-artery bypass. Doubts about his ability to exercise gradually diminished as he learned to take his pulse and to gauge his workout to stay within his prescribed training range, as determined by the number of heartbeats per minute. But perhaps most important were his colleagues in the program.

"Here were people who were much sicker than I, but they were out on the track every morning, working out with enthusiasm and vigor," he explained. "There is tremendous value in just talking to someone else who has been there before you: they know exactly how you feel, and can give invaluable advice and encouragement. And in the beginning, it is very comforting to know that there are doctors out on the track with you. I was actually afraid to walk fast or go up the stairs, but these fears disappeared when I had a doctor by my side. And after a few days, I could do it on my own."

ACTIVITY—THE KEY TO RECOVERY

A few decades ago, heart-attack patients were warned to take it easy for the rest of their lives. Many were forced to retire, especially if their jobs involved any sort of physical activity. Weeks of bed rest were usually advised, and even mild exercise was considered dangerous. Little wonder that so many heart-attack patients became cardiac cripples! This approach began to change in the 1950s. The late Dr. Paul Dudley White did much to dispel the notion that a heart attack meant the end of an active life when he told his most famous patient, President Eisenhower, to go back to work running the country, following a serious heart attack. Today, of course, the story is much different. Improved treatment, both in and out of the hospital, has greatly improved the chances of survival. In the large majority of cases, the heart muscle itself is not damaged severely enough to markedly impair the heart's ability to function. The major danger, at least for the first few days after a heart attack, is an unexpected disturbance in the heart's rhythm. This is why most heart-attack patients are continuously hooked up to an EKG monitor for the first few days. A number of drugs are now available to help prevent serious arrhythmias. There also are some instances in which the heart attack affects the natural pacemaker cells, resulting in a very slow heartbeat and inadequate pumping. In these cases, a temporary pacemaker may be needed until the heart's own conduction system recovers.

After the first few days, total bed rest is discouraged. In most cases, today's heart-attack patient is sitting up within a day or so, and walking about the hospital room as soon as medically sound: usually toward the end of the first week. Most heart-attack patients can now safely return home within two weeks. But it is the going-home phase that is hard for many to adjust to. There is a tendency for families to become overprotective and for the heart patient to let others wait on him. In the first few weeks after discharge, most heart patients can gradually increase their levels of activity, and by the end of two or three months, most find they can resume their normal activities. Of course, each patient is different, and some adjustments may have to be made, depending upon physical condition and the demands of job, family obligations, and other factors.

Ideally, the amount of physical activity you can undertake after a heart attack should be determined by your doctor on the basis of an exercise tolerance test. A growing number of hospitals are administering a modified exercise test before discharge; other physicians prefer to wait for a few more weeks. By undergoing an exercise test in a controlled medical setting, patient and doctor alike can know how much exercise can be undertaken without provoking symptoms or excessive fatigue. Using this as a guide, a specific exercise prescription can be made that will provide for a gradual increase in endurance and cardiovascular conditioning. (See "Exercise Conditioning: Getting Started the DUPAC Way," page 54–69.)

Of course, exercise is not the only fact of your life that should be scrutinized after a heart attack. If you are overweight, efforts should be made to gradually bring your weight to within normal levels. You should, however, avoid crash diets or very rapid weight loss. (See "Diet and the Heart," pages 95–145.) If you smoke, it is particularly imperative that you stop. A number of studies have demonstrated that continued smoking greatly increases the risk of subsequent heart attacks and sudden death. Stressful situations and emotional upsets should be avoided as much as possible. If stress is an unavoidable part of your daily life, then it may be worth your while to learn more effective coping techniques.

One question uppermost in the minds of many heart patients, but that many hesitate to discuss with their doctors, involves the resumption of sexual relations. DUPAC advises patients to approach sex in the same, positive manner as they approach any physical activity. Contrary to popular belief, sexual intercourse places only a modest work load on the heart. Unless you are so disabled that you have difficulty climbing a flight of stairs or walking a block, the heart is quite capable of meeting the work demands of sex. Most sexual dysfunction problems that occur following a heart attack are not due to cardiac limitations, but, instead, can be traced to psychological origins or are the result of drug treatments. Medications prescribed for high blood pressure sometimes cause impotence or reduced sexual desire. Since a satisfying, loving sexual relationship is such an important aspect of life, any difficulties in this area should be discussed with your doctor. The vast majority of heart patients are capable of normal sex lives; should problems occur, they almost always can be resolved.

Many heart-attack patients actually find they are healthier after recovery than they were before being stricken, especially if they modify things like overweight, smoking, or a sedentary life-style. But there also are people who require drugs or other treatment for high blood pressure, rhythm disturbances, or heart-muscle damage. If this is the case, it is vital that you be carefully evaluated and undergo appropriate treatment. The opportunity to fine-tune drug treatment is one of the advantages of a cardiac rehabilitation program such as DUPAC. Dosages can be adjusted, side effects observed, and other changes made that are not always possible during only periodic medical checkups.

SUMMING UP

A heart attack has a profound effect not only on the person who suffers it but also on family members, colleagues, and others. Major advances in the early treatment of heart attacks have greatly increased chances of survival.

But the quality of survival is also very important. Fortunately, most people who have heart attacks are able to resume a normal life-style. But to achieve this, it is important to determine functional capabilities and to learn how to maximize those capabilities safely and effectively. Carefully supervised exer-
·cise training, proper medical treatment of any continuing cardiovascular or other health problems, and emotional well-being all are important factors in high-quality survival.

Approaches to Treatment

Treating most forms of cardiovascular disease usually calls for a multifaceted approach that involves both life-style changes and medical therapy. The life-style changes—primarily increasing aerobic exercise, dietary modification, stress management, and stopping smoking—are discussed in other chapters. The major clinical treatments—drug therapy and surgery—will be reviewed here.

THE WORKUP

Obviously, the specific course of treatment must be determined by the type and extent of disease and other individual considerations—factors that can be ascertained only through a careful examination. This generally can be carried out in your doctor's office, although, depending upon the nature of the disorder, some components may be performed in a hospital or clinic setting.

The cardiovascular workup begins with a complete patient history. You will be questioned about any previous illnesses and treatments, the medical back-ground of family members, certain habits and other life-style factors, any symptoms you may be experiencing, and other aspects that may give your doctor further insight into your health status. (A sample of the Duke patient-history form is on pages 54–55.)

After the doctor has completed this history taking, he or she will move on to the physical examination. This will include the usual peering, listening, probing to determine the health of the various organ systems. Your eyes—the only place in the body where the small arteries and veins can be easily viewed —will be carefully examined for any signs of blood-vessel damage. If there is suspected cardiovascular disease, particular attention will be paid to the heart. You may be asked to assume several positions while your doctor listens to the heart sounds through a stethoscope. A resting electrocardiogram will be done to study the electrical activity of the heart and to detect signs of heart-muscle damage, enlargement, or other abnormalities. (Contrary to popular belief, the EKG does not measure the heart's pumping capability.) A chest X-ray film may be made. Several blood-pressure measurements may be taken, at various times during the examination. Circulation to the legs and feet may be studied, and your doctor will note any signs of edema (swelling caused by a buildup of body fluids, which may result from a variety of factors, including many that are unrelated to heart disease).

In addition to a careful physical examination, a number of laboratory studies will be required. These will include blood and urine tests to determine such things as levels of cholesterol and of triglycerides, uric acid, and numerous other biochemical components.

An exercise-tolerance test may be performed, either in the doctor's office or, more likely, in a hospital out-patient clinic. There are now a number of variations on exercise testing, and the type performed depends upon the nature and extent of suspected disease. The most common is still the simple treadmill or bicycle exercise test, which involves exercising while under constant electrographic monitoring. This test reveals how much work the heart is capable of; it may also detect certain abnormalities, but with varying degrees of accuracy. Simple pulmonary tests to study how well the lungs are functioning also may be performed during a treadmill exercise test.

More sophisticated exercise tests that use an array of nuclear studies are being used increasingly to gather information about the heart's functional capability. The nuclear studies, in which a substance containing radioactive particles is injected into the heart's circulatory system and then followed by special cameras or tracing devices, provides valuable information about the structure and function of the heart. One of the most revealing measurements of the heart's functional capability is the ejection fraction. Each time the heart beats, the left ventricle contracts and pumps a portion of its blood into the circulatory system. The ejection fraction measures the completeness of the left ventricle's emptying. A normal, healthy heart can empty 50 to 60 percent—stated as an ejection fraction of 50 or 60—of the blood from the left ventricle, while a sick heart may empty only 20 percent or even less.

There may be instances in which it is desirable to monitor the heart for an extended period and during a variety of normal activities. To do this, you may be asked to wear a twenty-four-hour Holter monitor, a portable electrographic device. Electrodes are attached to specific points of the chest; the EKG device is contained in a small cassette-like box that can be carried at the waist or from a shoulder strap. The patient keeps a diary of activities and occurrences of symptoms or unusual events while wearing the monitor. For example, if chest pain occurs, the patient would press a button on the monitor and also record the symptom and time in the twenty-four-hour diary. The doctor can later examine the EKG tracings and the diary to get a better picture of how the heart is functioning.

In some types of heart disease, particularly disorders of the heart valves, echocardiography may be employed. This technique, also known as sonography, uses sound waves to map internal structures. The principle is the same as that employed in sonar. Sound waves are beamed at a structure, and their reflection provides information about size, shape, internal cavities, and other physical characteristics. Echocardiography can provide an accurate map of the heart and its various parts, and by observing the echocardiograms in motion, doctors can study the action of the heart valves as the blood is moved from chamber to chamber. Echocardiography is a safe, painless procedure that can be performed in an out-patient clinic.

If these various noninvasive tests do not provide adequate information about the suspected heart disease, further examinations that enable a doctor to actually probe the inside of the heart and the coronary vessels may be required. The most common of these invasive examinations—so named because they involve going into the body—is coronary angiography. In this examination, a long, flexible catheter is threaded through the circulatory system after entering through an incision made either in the arm, leg, or both, and finally moving into the heart chambers and coronary arteries. A radiopaque substance, which makes the blood vessels visible on X-ray film or a fluoroscopic screen, is injected through the catheter. By studying the X-ray films taken during coronary angiography, a doctor can detect blocked or seriously narrowed coronary arteries—a key factor in deciding whether a patient is a candidate for coronary-artery bypass surgery. In fact, coronary angiography is always done before a bypass operation. Angiography is performed in a hospital setting and usually requires an overnight stay for observation. Several hundred thousand of these examinations are performed annually in the United States, and in the vast majority, there are no complications. In a small percentage of patients, however, there is a risk of complication, including a heart attack. Complications are most likely to occur in patients who already have serious coronary-artery disease.

There are numerous other cardiovascular examinations that may be performed, especially after a heart attack. Some of these assess the extent of damage; others may measure or monitor heart rhythm and blood pressure.

TYPES OF TREATMENT

The large majority of heart patients can be treated conservatively with drugs and life-style modification. Surgery, such as coronary-artery bypass and valve replacement, is usually reserved for those patients who can benefit more from an operative procedure than from drugs or more conservative approaches. Although a complete discussion of what is involved in the various approaches to treating heart disease is beyond the scope of this book, the general principles in treating the major forms of heart disease are outlined below.

Coronary-Artery Disease

People with coronary-artery disease are often undergoing treatment for other conditions, such as high blood pressure, high blood cholesterol, diabetes, gout, or obesity. Some of these may be directly related to the heart disease; others may be predisposing conditions. The treatment for some, particularly high blood pressure, may even be combined with the treatment for coronary disease.

There are several classes of drugs that may be prescribed for coronary disease, especially if there are symptoms such as chest pain (angina pectoris), shortness of breath, or irregular heart rhythm. These drug classes include:

Nitrates. These are among the oldest drugs to treat angina; they have been used for nearly one hundred years and still are the most commonly prescribed drug for angina. Nitrates now come in several forms: as nitroglycerine tablets, to be placed under the tongue to bring relief during an attack; as long-acting pills or capsules to be taken regularly to prevent chest pain; or as a salve, ointment, or medicated disk to be absorbed through the skin, also to prevent anginal attacks. The nitrates work by widening the blood vessels and by a complicated mechanism that increases the blood supply to the heart, and perhaps by other mechanisms that are still not fully understood. People who suffer from angina should carry their nitroglycerine with them at all times, and also should learn to use it to prevent attacks by taking it in anticipation of circumstances—physical exertion or emotional stress, for example—that may provoke an attack. Since nitroglycerine deteriorates in warm, moist places, it should not be stored in a bathroom medicine chest or carried in a pocket close to the body. Make sure, too, that you replenish your supply periodically.

Beta-adrenergic-blocking drugs. These drugs, commonly called simply beta blockers, were introduced over a decade ago and are now widely used to treat coronary disease, high blood pressure, and certain disorders of heart rhythm. They also may be prescribed following a heart attack in an attempt to prevent future infarctions. Beta blockers work by slowing the heart rate and reducing the force of contractions, thus lowering the heart muscle's need for oxygen. They also lower blood pressure. They may be used alone or in conjunction with nitrates and other antianginal drugs.

Calcium-blocking drugs. These are the newest class of antianginal drugs. They are particularly effective in controlling the type of angina associated with spasm of the coronary arteries. They work by reducing the amount of calcium that enters the muscle cells of the coronary vessels. All muscles require calcium in order to contract; by reducing the amount available to the coronary blood vessels, it is possible to prevent muscle spasms, which narrow the artery and reduce the blood supply to the heart muscle.

High Blood Pressure

Over the past three decades, a number of drugs to lower high blood pressure have been developed, thus revolutionizing the treatment of this exceedingly common condition. Until the development of these drugs, the major treatments were weight loss, salt restriction (which at times meant living on a diet of rice and fruit), and surgery (which was not very effective). Today, most cases of high blood pressure can be controlled by drugs, which may be prescribed singly or in combination. Weight reduction is still an important factor for those who are overweight, and lowering salt consumption is still advocated by most doctors even if the blood pressure can be controlled by drugs. By reducing salt intake, the drugs may be made even more effective in controlling blood pressure, meaning that a lower dosage may be prescribed. This reduces the chances of adverse side effects from the drugs. Other measures, such as stress management and exercise, also may play a role in helping to lower high blood pressure.

The classes of drugs used to treat high blood pressure include:

Diuretics. These drugs, commonly referred to as water pills, lower blood pressure by reducing the body's sodium and water volume. There are several kinds of diuretics, but the type most commonly prescribed for hypertension are the thiazide diuretics. Treatment for mild to moderate hypertension usually begins with a thiazide diuretic; if this fails to lower the blood pressure, other drugs may be added.

Beta-blocking agents. These are the same drugs that are often used to treat angina or given following a heart attack. It is not fully understood how they lower blood pressure, although it is generally agreed that they somehow work through the nervous system to reduce the constriction of the blood vessels. A beta blocker may be prescribed with a thiazide diuretic or alone as an initial treatment of high blood pressure when a diuretic is not advisable.

Vasodilators. These drugs act by relaxing the muscles in the blood-vessel walls, causing the vessels to widen, or dilate. This lets the blood flow through them with less resistance. Vasodilators are often prescribed along with a diuretic or a beta blocker.

Centrally acting drugs. These antihypertensive agents work through the sympathetic nervous system, which controls involuntary muscle action. They decrease the heart rate and lower the amount of blood that is pumped with each beat. They are usually prescribed along with a thiazide diuretic.

Alpha-adrenergic-blocking drugs. These drugs act by blocking some of the nerve impulses that control blood-vessel constriction, thus widening the vessels. They are often given with a diuretic.

Angiotensin-converting-enzyme (ACE) inhibitors. These drugs are the newest class of antihypertensives. Also referred to as rinin-axis blockers, they act by interfering with the formation of angiotensin, a powerful vessel-constricting substance. They also lower the body's ability to retain salt and water.

Although most cases of high blood pressure can be controlled by prescribing one or more antihypertensive drugs, these agents do not cure the disease. Once you stop taking the drugs, blood pressure tends to go back up, sometimes to even higher levels than before. Therefore, it is important to continue taking the drugs even if the blood pressure returns to normal, and to have your pressure checked periodically by your doctor. If side effects do occur—some of the more common are dizziness or fainting when standing, unusual tiredness, depression, and loss of sexual desire or function—they should be reported promptly to your doctor. In most cases, the side effects can be eliminated or minimized by adjusting the dosage or changing to a different drug.

Elevated Blood Lipids

High blood cholesterol is usually treated by lowering consumption of fats, particularly the fats in animal and dairy products. If diet fails to adequately lower the blood lipids, or if the patient has a hereditary disorder called familial hypercholesterolemia, which carries a very high risk of an early heart attack, drugs to lower the blood lipids may be prescribed. Some of these drugs act by increasing the excretion of fats from the intestinal tract; the mechanism of action for others is not fully understood.

Congestive Heart Failure

Also referred to as cardiac failure, this disorder does not indicate that the heart is failing to beat, as is popularly thought; rather, it is characterized by an enlarged heart with a progressive pumping impairment. The earlier this condition is diagnosed and treatment started, the better the prognosis. If the cause is hypertension, lowering the blood pressure will also aid in the treatment of cardiac failure. Cardiac failure also may result from a heart attack; in these cases, treatment will be incorporated into the coronary care program. Other causes include disease of the heart muscle (cardiomyopathy) and diseased heart valves. Weight loss, salt restriction, and a program of exercise and rest also may be recommended, depending upon individual circumstances.

Several classes of drugs are used to treat congestive heart disease; these include:

Cardiac glycosides or digitalis. Digitalis, originally derived from the foxglove plant, is one of the oldest heart drugs. Centuries ago, it was a popular folk remedy for dropsy (edema), and early physicians recognized its value in treating congestive failure. Today it is still the most commonly used drug for this disease, although now it is usually given in combination with a diuretic. It acts by strengthening the heart's contractility. It also has a mild diuretic effect, and it is used to treat certain types of arrhythmias that may accompany cardiac failure.

Diuretics. These drugs increase the body's excretion of sodium, thereby reducing the fluid volume and, indirectly, the work load of the heart. They may be used alone for mild congestive disease, or may be given in conjunction with digitalis.

Angiotensin-converting-enzyme (ACE) inhibitors. These drugs, which may be used to treat hypertension that cannot be controlled by other agents, are also useful in treating congestive heart disease. They act by widening the blood vessels and thereby easing the heart's work load.

Cardiac Arrhythmias

There are many kinds of disturbance of heart rhythm; treatment depends upon the type of arrhythmia. Some of the more common drugs used in treating arrhythmias include:

Quinidine. This drug, an alkaloid derived from cinchona-tree bark, acts by reducing the excitability of the heart muscle, thereby slowing the heart rate. It also reduces the amount of blood pumped from the heart.

Procainamide. The antiarrhythmic actions of this drug are similar to those of quinidine; the two agents are sometimes used interchangeably.

Digitalis. Antiarrhythmic drugs derived from digitalis glycosides may be prescribed to treat the rapid heartbeats (e.g., atrial flutter or fibrillation, supraventricular tachycardia, or ventricular premature beats) that may occur with congestive heart failure.

Beta-adrenergic-blocking drugs. Beta blockers—commonly used to treat hypertension and angina—also have an important antiarrhythmic effect. They slow the heartbeat, so they may be prescribed for a variety of tachycardias (rapid heart rhythms). They also may be used to treat the palpitations that sometimes occur in mitral-valve prolapse.

Lidocaine. This drug may be administered to treat the severe ventricular arrhythmias that sometimes occur following a heart attack or during surgery.

Calcium-blocking agents. These drugs, which also are used to treat angina, may be administered to treat serious ventricular tachycardias.

Atropine. This is an anticholinergic drug, meaning it prevents the transmission of certain nerve impulses, resulting in an increased heart rate. Atropine may be prescribed in some cases of bradycardia (slow heartbeat), which may accompany some heart attacks.

There are a number of other drugs, with miscellaneous actions, used to treat cardiac arrhythmias. Care must be taken in administering many of these antiarrhythmic drugs, because the drugs themselves may provoke serious disturbances in the heart's rhythm. Digitalis is a case in point; even a very small overdose can cause serious upset in heart rhythm.

Artificial pacemakers may be implanted to control arrhythmias that cannot be managed with drugs. They may be used temporarily after a heart attack or permanently in the case of fast beats followed by very slow ones, resulting in an inadequate output of blood from the heart.

Heart-Valve Disease

The heart has four sets of valves that control the flow of blood from one chamber to another and, finally, from the heart into the aorta. Valvular disease is not as common today as in the past, largely because two of the major causes are now better controlled, namely rheumatic fever and syphilis. Some valvular disorders, particularly mitral-valve prolapse—a common condition in which one of the two mitral leaflets fails to close completely—are relatively minor and usually require little or no treatment. However, if the valvular disease progresses to the point that the flow of blood through the heart is seriously impaired, treatment may be required. Drugs to control cardiac arrhythmias may be prescribed if palpitations occur, as is sometimes the case with mitral-valve disease. Anticoagulants also may be prescribed to prevent the formation of clots. If breathlessness and fluid retention (edema) occur, a diuretic may be prescribed. Since people with valvular disease have an increased risk of a serious heart infection—bacterial endocarditis—antibiotics should be taken before any surgical or dental procedure that may release bacteria into the bloodstream. Avoiding strenuous activities and taking frequent rest periods during the day also may be recommended for people with heart-valve disease.

If the heart's function becomes seriously impaired, surgery to replace the diseased valve with an artificial one may be in order. These artificial valves are constructed either from animal parts or from plastic and metal. While artificial valves may not be as efficient as the natural ones, they have enabled many people once doomed to increasing disability to again lead relatively active, normal lives.

CORONARY-ARTERY BYPASS SURGERY

No discussion of the modern treatment of heart disease can be complete without at least a brief review of coronary-artery bypass surgery. Each year, more than 170,000 people undergo bypass surgery; in some areas, it is now the most frequently performed operation.

In brief, a coronary-artery bypass involves taking healthy blood vessels from one part of the body (usually veins in the leg) and grafting them onto the heart's surface to bypass one or more clogged coronary arteries. This increases the blood flow to the heart muscle normally served by the diseased artery. The operation takes four to six hours; during that time, circulation is maintained with the aid of a heart-lung machine. Following the surgery, patients spend a few days in an intensive-care unit, and if all goes well a few days in a regular coronary unit and then a week or so in a regular hospital setting. Most bypass patients are discharged from the hospital within ten days to two weeks of the surgery.

Coronary-artery bypass is most commonly recommended for patients who have severe disabling angina that cannot be controlled by drugs, exercise conditioning, or other conservative treatments. It is also the treatment of choice for patients who have a severely diseased left main coronary artery. Although some disagreement persists among cardiologists as to other clear indications for coronary bypass, there is increasing evidence that it may prevent a heart attack or prolong life in people with three (and in some instances even two) seriously diseased coronary arteries.

There are, of course, some people with disease falling into these categories who still are not good candidates for surgery because of age, poor health, or other medical problems. It should be noted also that the operation itself involves a degree of risk. But despite these drawbacks, the majority of people who undergo coronary bypasses experience relief from angina and other symptoms, and many find they have considerably more energy.

Although most bypass patients experience favorable results, it would be a mistake for them to think the operation has cured their underlying heart disease. The new grafts appear to become diseased even more rapidly than the natural coronary arteries; therefore, it is particularly important to reduce or remove as many risk factors (e.g., smoking, elevated blood cholesterol, stress, etc.) as possible. Some preliminary studies suggest that taking small doses of aspirin (one-half tablet a day) may help keep the grafted vessels from closing. Exercise is also thought to be an important preventive measure for the bypass patient.

A LOOK AT THE FUTURE

Research is constantly refining present treatments and developing new ones that promise an even brighter outlook for heart patients. Some of these new procedures are technically still listed as experimental but already are being done with marked success at a number of medical centers. Balloon angioplasty is an example. This procedure involves threading a specially designed balloon catheter into a diseased coronary artery and gradually inflating the balloon to flatten the fatty obstruction. In the first three thousand patients to undergo this procedure, 60 percent were considered successful. (In 29 percent the obstructed areas could not be crossed with the balloon catheter, and in 11 percent the obstruction could not be flattened.) Patients in whom angioplasty does not work may still have to undergo bypass surgery, but the 60 percent in whom it is successful have been treated with a much simpler and less costly procedure.

Other promising areas now under investigation include the use of lasers to dissolve the fatty deposits from both coronary arteries and blood vessels elsewhere in the body. Laser surgery, which uses concentrated light sources instead of the traditional scalpel, is being used increasingly in a number of operations; many authorities feel that it also has great promise in treating some forms of coronary disease.

SUMMING UP

Most heart patients can live with their disease by following conservative measures: life-style changes to lower cardiovascular risk factors, exercise conditioning, and drug therapy as indicated. Some problems may require more aggressive treatment, such as surgery to replace diseased heart valves or to bypass diseased coronary arteries. There is little doubt that the considerable advances in treating cardiovascular diseases over the past few decades has contributed to the declining death rate from heart attacks. Further, ongoing research promises even more progress in the not too distant future.

Exercise and the Heart

The idea that exercise is good for body and mind is hardly new. In 300 B.C., Hippocrates said, "Speaking generally, all parts of the body which have a function, if used in moderation and exercised in labors in which each is accustomed, thereby become healthy, well developed and age more slowly; but if unused and left idle, they become liable to disease, defective in growth and age quickly."

It is only relatively recently in the history of man, however, that lack of exercise has become a health problem for large segments of the population. Before the industrial revolution, only the very rich and a few others were privileged enough not to have to live by hard physical labor. Almost every task, from washing clothes to tilling the earth and soldiering involved hard work. Today, thanks to the mechanization of almost every task, very few people exert enough physical effort in their jobs to remain physically fit. There are, of course, a few exceptions: postmen who walk many miles delivering mail and dockworkers are two examples that have been studied to see if their health statistics are comparable to the rest of the population. Those studies have found that people whose jobs demand physical exertion enjoy a lower-than-average incidence of heart attacks. Similarly, a study involving several thousand college alumni found that those whose recreational activities were the equivalent of jogging twenty-five miles a week also had a low incidence of heart disease. These students do not prove that exercise can prevent a heart attack, but there is ample evidence that the right kind of exercise done on a regular basis benefits not only the heart but the entire body. It also produces enhanced psychological well-being.

THE FITNESS BOOM

In recent years, millions of Americans seem to have gotten the message that regular exercise is important to health and well-being. This has given birth to the so-called fitness boom. Today it is estimated that some 20 million Americans jog regularly and millions more play tennis or other racket sports, swim, bicycle, or participate in some form of aerobic exercise. Dr. R. Sanders Williams, Director of Research for DUPAC, explains the reasons behind this increased interest in fitness by saying, "The most common motivations are likely to be twofold: 'I feel better when I exercise,' and 'Regular exercise is going to help me be healthier and live longer.'" Dr. Lenore R. Zohman, a New York City expert in exercise physiology and cardiopulmonary rehabilitation, adds a third motivation: "Many people exercise because they want to stay trim and look more attractive."

Although millions of formerly sedentary people are now exercising, it would be wrong to give the impression that this has become a universal trend. The mostly sedentary still outnumber the active, and many people who consider themselves physically active do not exercise sufficiently to gain the benefits of cardiovascular conditioning. Technically, physical fitness is defined as having enough endurance or stamina to exercise at or near your biological potential. This is usually expressed in terms of METS, which are multiples of resting metabolism. Even when you are at rest, your body requires a certain amount of minimal energy to sustain life: breathing, circulation, digestion, and other vital functions. The number of multiples above your resting metabolism that you can comfortably sustain is a standard measurement of fitness. Well-conditioned athletes can sustain twenty METS, or twenty times their minimum energy expenditure. Physically fit people can usually sustain ten to fifteen METS, while those who are sedentary often cannot exercise above five METS, even though they may be otherwise healthy. (People with serious heart or lung disease may be similarly limited in their ability to exercise.) If you are in poor physical condition, you will not be able to climb a flight of stairs or run a block to catch a bus without feeling winded, even though you may not have any evidence of heart disease. In contrast, if you are physically fit, you will be able to jog, play tennis, bicycle, or engage in other vigorous activities without becoming quickly fatigued, and also without putting as much demand on your heart. What's more, you will sleep better, have better control of your appetite, and have an improved disposition. But to achieve these benefits, you need to engage in the right kinds of aerobic exercise—that is, a physical activity in which the large muscles of the body require an increased and sustained supply of oxygen—on a regular, progressive basis.

BENEFITS OF CARDIOVASCULAR CONDITIONING

The body—particularly the heart, lungs, and blood vessels—undergoes several important changes when a sedentary person undertakes an aerobic exercise program. At first, the effort may produce fatigue after only a few minutes. The heart rate may quickly rise to your maximum training level, and you may feel short of breath or winded. After a week or two of gradual exercise training, however, you will notice that your endurance has increased: you are able to exercise longer, your heart rate is not as high, and you don't feel as out of breath. In this short a time, your body already is showing the benefits of exercise training. In simplified terms, here's what is happening.

During any aerobic exercise—walking, jogging, bicycling, swimming, and so forth—a large number of muscles are called into action. These muscles, in order to continue working at a steady pace, require extra oxygen. This oxygen is delivered by an increased flow of blood through the body. Instead of pumping about six quarts of blood in a minute (the average cardiac output for a sedentary man weighing about 150 pounds), the heart is called upon to pump more than four times that much—about twenty-five quarts—during maximum exercise. To do this, the heart has to beat faster and also pump more blood with each beat. To further ensure that the muscles get the oxygen they need, some blood will be diverted from the kidneys, liver, intestines, and other internal organs, and instead will circulate to the muscles. At the same time, the blood vessels that supply the muscles will widen, or dilate. In all, the blood supply to the muscles will increase from about 20 percent of the six quarts pumped per minute during rest to 90 percent of the twenty-five quarts pumped during maximum exercise.

During exercise conditioning, two important changes in oxygen transport and utilization take place: the blood increases its ability to carry oxygen, and even more important, the well-trained muscles are capable of extracting more oxygen from the blood. During rest, only about 30 percent of the oxygen in the blood is actually extracted as it circulates through the body. During vigorous exercise, several chemical changes take place that speed up metabolism and consume more oxygen—over 75 percent of what is available—from the blood. This is known as maximal oxygen uptake, and it determines the limits of your endurance. An increase in maximal oxygen uptake is important, because it means the body is making more efficient use of the available oxygen and is not putting so much demand on the heart.

The heart muscle (myocardium) itself also benefits from exercise conditioning. Like any muscle, the myocardium grows stronger the more it is exercised. As it grows stronger, the heart muscle can pump more blood with each beat and can therefore deliver the needed oxygen-rich blood to the body with fewer beats. This is why the resting heart rate of a conditioned athlete is often much lower than that of the average person. Thus, if exercise conditioning lowers the average resting heart rate by ten beats per minute, over a year's time this would total 5 million fewer beats per minute. This does not necessarily mean that a slower heart rate will result in a longer life, but it is obvious that a well-conditioned heart does not have to work as hard to pump the same amount of blood. The slower heart rate also means that the cardiac muscle is able to use oxygen more efficiently. The heart-muscle contraction that accompanies each beat momentarily interrupts the flow of blood through the coronary vessels. If there is more time between heartbeats—as is the case with a lowered heart rate—then the interruptions are fewer and the heart muscle is better nourished. Therefore, cardiovascular conditioning can, to a degree, compensate for the effects of arteries that have been narrowed by coronary disease.

EFFECTS ON BLOOD PRESSURE

There is no definite proof that exercise alone will lower high resting blood pressure, although a number of studies have found that some hypertensives undergoing exercise conditioning achieve a moderate reduction. This is not a universal finding, however, and exercise does not seem to affect normal blood pressure. Even so, there are some people with mild hypertension for whom exercise, especially when it is combined with weight control and reduced intake of sodium, is sufficient to return the blood pressure to normal. The reasons for this are unknown; most experts think it is probably a combination of factors.

EFFECTS ON WEIGHT

People who undertake exercise conditioning usually lose some weight, even though they may continue to eat their regular diet or even more food than usual. There are several reasons for this. Any physical activity consumes calories, and the more intense the activity, the more calories are required. (See Table of Energy Expenditure of Various Types of Exercise.) Thus, if you burn up an extra 350 calories per day—the average energy consumption of a

ENERGY EXPENDITURE
OF VARIOUS TYPES OF EXERCISE

Activity	Calories Used (per minute)
Walking (1 mph)	2–2.5
Walking (2 mph)	2.5–4
Walking (3 mph) or cycling (6 mph)	4–5
Walking (3.5 mph), cycling (8 mph), tennis doubles or vigorous dancing	5–6
Walking (4 mph), cycling (10 mph), swimming (breaststroke, 1 mph), ice or roller skating	6–7
Walking (5 mph), cycling (11 mph), tennis singles, swimming (breaststroke, 1.6 mph)	7–8
Jogging (5 mph), cycling (12 mph), mountain hiking, swimming (sidestroke, 1 mph)	8–10
Jogging (5.5 mph), cycling (13 mph), swimming (backstroke, 1.6 mph), squash or handball	10–11
Running (8 mph), rowing, cross-country skiing, competitive handball or squash	11–12

35–40-minute conditioning workout or the equivalent of jogging 5 miles in 40 minutes or walking 3.5 miles in an hour—you will lose a pound in about ten days. This is assuming you do not alter your food consumption. If you are on a weight-reduction diet, you will lose unwanted pounds more rapidly; if you are of normal weight, you can increase the amount you eat without gaining.

In addition to helping you lose weight, there is evidence that exercise will help maintain ideal weight once you stop dieting. Recent studies have found that body metabolism is somewhat slowed during weight loss, especially if the diet involves extreme reduction in calories for a more rapid weight loss. Just as the body adjusts to near starvation by slowing down to conserve energy, our metabolic thermostat is reset at a lower level during crash dieting. This explains in part why so many people lose a lot of weight initially when going on a diet, but when metabolism changes, the weight loss becomes slower, even though the same number of calories are being consumed. In other words, the body has readjusted its metabolism to get by on less food. This is not as likely to happen if the weight-loss program provides for a moderate reduction in calories and an increase in physical activity. The muscles will become more proficient in utilizing the stores of body fat, weight will fall, and the reserves of fat will be diminished. Since the percentage of body fat changes with improved muscle tone, well-conditioned people look trimmer and are less flabby even though they may weigh the same as more sedentary people.

EFFECT ON CHOLESTEROL AND OTHER BLOOD FATS

A high level of blood cholesterol is among the major risk factors for a heart attack. But the total cholesterol is not the entire story; the type of cholesterol is also important. (See "Diet and the Heart," pages 95–145.) Several studies have found that people who engage in regular vigorous exercise have an increase in HDL (high-density-lipoprotein) cholesterol, which, as noted earlier, is considered protective against the buildup of fatty deposits in the coronary arteries. Some studies also have found that exercise conditioning may lower total cholesterol and triglycerides, but this is most likely to happen as a result of weight loss and dietary changes, rather than because of the exercise itself.

PSYCHOLOGICAL EFFECTS

Invariably, when formerly sedentary people undertake an exercise conditioning program, they are surprised at how much better they feel, not only physically but also emotionally. They are more relaxed, are better able to handle stress, and have a renewed sense of well-being. They talk about a new kind of "high" they get from exercise, and some seem to become addicted: if they can't exercise for a day or two, they complain of feeling jittery and on edge, as if they were experiencing withdrawal symptoms. Biochemical analyses of exercisers have found that they have a high level of endorphins—naturally occurring body chemicals that can, among other things, blunt pain and produce euphoria similar to that of morphine. In short, when runners talk about being addicted to the activity, there is considerable truth to the statement. But, unlike so many addictions (smoking, alcohol, and drugs, to name a few), getting hooked on exercise has few harmful effects unless carried to extremes.

Recent research also has confirmed that exercise conditioning can improve psychological functioning. For example, Duke research involving thirty-two healthy middle-aged adults studied six mood states and found marked differences between the active and the inactive. Sixteen of the participants underwent a ten-week exercise conditioning program, while the other sixteen carried on as usual. All of the participants underwent physical and psychological testing both before and after the ten-week program. At the end of the ten weeks, all of the exercise group showed improved physical condition, a result that had been expected. But the exercisers showed equally pronounced changes in the psychological testing, which covered tension/anxiety, depression/dejection, anger/hostility, vigor/activity, fatigue/inertia, and confusion/bewilderment. "In virtually every comparison," the researchers reported, "the exercise group changed in the desired direction, while the control group remained the same or actually got worse." (See "Stress, Personality, and Heart Disease," pages 146–65.)

ADDITIONAL BENEFITS OF EXERCISE

A number of other benefits of regular exercise have been documented. These include:

Reduced danger from blood clots. Recent studies have found that exercise may affect the body's ability to produce or dissolve blood clots. The formation of clots within blood vessels is thought to be an important step in several disease processes, including atherosclerosis (development of fatty deposits along the artery lining), stroke, and heart attacks. Regular exercise appears to reduce the danger of blood clots in two ways: It enhances the body's ability to dissolve clots, a process known as fibrinolysis. It also may reduce the degree to which platelets (tiny corpuscles in the blood) adhere to sites of damage on the inside of blood vessels. A number of recent studies have focused on the question of platelet stickiness or clumping, particularly at the site of an injury to the artery lining. Preliminary evidence indicates that such platelet clumping may set in motion the atherosclerotic process.

Response to insulin. Regular exercise improves the ability of cells to utilize insulin, the hormone that enables the body to metabolize glucose (blood sugar). This is particularly important in diabetics, and overweight people who may have a tendency to diabetes. Diabetics who exercise regularly have better control of their blood sugar. In fact, many adult-onset diabetics are able to reduce or even discontinue their medication after undergoing exercise conditioning and weight control.

SUMMING UP

Although exercise is not the cure-all that some enthusiasts would have us believe, there are a number of documented benefits to be gained from exercise conditioning. A word of caution, however: Before undertaking an exercise program, be sure to read the following chapter, "Exercise Conditioning: Getting Started the DUPAC Way." This is particularly important if you have any symptoms of heart disease or have had a heart attack. It is also important if you are physically inactive and fall into any of the high-risk groups for a heart attack.

Exercise Conditioning: Getting Started the DUPAC Way

By now, you know the many benefits of exercise conditioning; the question is how to go about getting started. Unfortunately, there is no one answer that applies to everyone. A good deal depends upon your physical condition and age. Do you have coronary disease or some other heart disorder? Are you overweight? Do you have arthritis or other joint or muscle problems? The accompanying Sample Medical Questionnaire, which all DUPAC participants complete before starting a conditioning program, indicates the kind of health information that is important.

THE MEDICAL CHECKUP

Ideally, an inactive, sedentary person contemplating starting an exercise program should have a medical checkup first. This should include an examination of the cardiovascular system: an electrocardiogram, blood-pressure measurement, evaluation of cholesterol and triglycerides, and for some individuals an exercise stress, or tolerance, test. A more extensive workup may be indicated for people who have had a heart attack, suffer angina when exercising, or have other symptoms of heart disease.

Sample Medical Questionnaire

History #: _____

Name:_____/_____/_____ Date:__/__/__
　　　　(Last)　　　　(First)　　　　(MI)

Sex: _____ Date of Birth: __/__/__ Race: _____ Height: _____

Occupation: _____ Work status: full time, part time, unemployed, disabled, sick leave, retired

Comments:_____

Summary:_____

_____

_____

_____

Problem List: (coronary artery disease, angina, heart attack, hypertension, obesity,
valvular disease, hyperlipidemia, congestive heart disease,
arrhythmia, pulmonary embolus, transient ischemic attacks, stroke,
claudication, chronic obstructive pulmonary disease, depression)

1)_____   6)_____
2)_____   7)_____
3)_____   8)_____
4)_____   9)_____
5)_____   10)_____

If chest pain: Angina (typical, atypical, nonangina)
  nocturnal: Yes No   Average frequency per week: _____
  Course (improving, stable, progressive)
If heart attack, date:_____ Complication: Yes No
  Work status prior to heart attack
Medications:

  _____   _____

  _____   _____

  _____   _____

  _____

Risk Factor History
  Smoking: History of smoking: Yes No   Number per Day:_____
    Currently smoking: Yes No   If stopped, how many months ago _____
  Hypertension: Yes No   Age at onset _____
    End organ damage_____
  Glucose intolerance: Yes No   Diabetes: Yes No   Age at onset _____
    Insulin dependent: Yes No   Retinopathy, nephropathy, neuropathy
  Activity: Miles walked/wk:_____   Miles jogged/wk:_____

  _____

Family History: (before age 65, if yes, enter age of onset)

	Coronary disease	Stroke	Hypertension	Diabetes
Father	Yes/No/Age____	N____	N____	N____
Mother	Yes/No/Age____	N____	N____	N____
Brother	Yes/No/Age____	N____	N____	N____
Sister	Yes/No/Age____	N____	N____	N____

Weight: now_____ one yr. ago_____ age 18_____ age 21_____

The question of who should have an exercise stress test is still open to
debate. The American Heart Association's Committee on Exercise recommends that anyone over the age of thirty-five who has been relatively seden-

tary undergo an exercise stress test before taking up exercise conditioning. This is based on the knowledge that about 10 percent of all men over the age of thirty-five who are ostensibly normal have some form of hidden heart disease. The American Medical Association's Committee on Physical Fitness and Exercise recommends that people between the ages of thirty and thirty-nine should have a checkup within three months before starting an exercise program and that the checkup include a resting electrocardiogram. After the age of forty, this group recommends, everyone undergo an exercise stress test before starting an exercise program.

In recent years, a growing number of medical consumers have questioned the need for exercise testing on a routine basis in people with no symptoms. The magazine *Runners World*, for example, urges its readers to "Bypass the Stress Test," and there are many people over the age of thirty-five or forty who have safely undergone exercise conditioning without an exercise test. To enroll in DUPAC, an exercise test is administered to all participants in the medical program, since most of these are heart patients, and exercise testing is always indicated for anyone who has had a heart attack or been diagnosed as having coronary-artery disease or any other cardiovascular disorder. But basically healthy people under the age of forty who are enrolling as part of the general conditioning program need not take an exercise test unless they fall into a high-risk category. Specifically, this would include people with any such symptom as chest pain or irregular heartbeats, people with high blood pressure or high blood cholesterol, those who are markedly overweight or smoke, or anyone with a parent who had a heart attack before the age of fifty.

To undergo an exercise tolerance test, you will be asked to walk on a treadmill or pedal a bicycle while undergoing continuous EKG monitoring. This involves having electrodes from an electrocardiographic monitor attached to specific places on your chest throughout the test. Your blood pressure while resting will be measured before beginning, and then intermittently throughout the test and again after it is completed. You should wear comfortable, loose-fitting exercise clothes and sneakers. As the test progresses, the speed and intensity of the exercise will be increased, usually at one to three-minute intervals. As the work demands on the heart increase, it will beat faster and blood pressure will rise. The test will continue until a point of exhaustion is reached or until you achieve a predetermined heart rate. It may be stopped if chest pain occurs, you feel weak or faint, or there are abnormal changes in heart rhythm or in the electrocardiogram, or any other indications of exercise intolerance.

People who have a narrowing of one or more of the coronary arteries may have changes on the electrocardiogram as the heart is forced to work harder. This is because the heart muscle that is ordinarily nourished by the diseased vessels will be deprived of oxygen, and this lack of oxygen (ischemia) usually produces changes in the electrical conduction system of the heart—changes that are often detectable in the electrocardiographic tracings. But, as a diagnostic tool, the exercise test is not 100 percent accurate; some people with completely normal hearts will, for unexplained reasons, have abnormal electrocardiograms, while some who do have heart disease may have a normal test. This happens often enough that we cannot completely trust the results, which limits its use as a diagnostic tool. Even so, the exercise test helps identify people who may be at a high risk for a heart attack. In people who have no symptoms, for example, an abnormal stress test may indicate there is indeed hidden heart disease, and further testing may be in order. Although the test cannot predict who will or will not have a heart attack, studies have found that people who are able to achieve a high work level during an exercise test, despite extensive coronary disease, are less likely to have a heart attack than those who must stop at a low level even though they have a normal electrocardiogram.

Perhaps the most important role of the exercise test, however, is in providing information about how well the heart is functioning. In designing an exercise conditioning program, such as DUPAC, it is vital to know just how much work the heart is capable of performing. "In this sense," explains DUPAC's Program Director, Paul Koisch, "we are more interested in how well the heart is functioning as opposed to how sick it is." From this perspective, the exercise test is used as a basis for determining the parameters for an exercise conditioning program that is designed to meet individual differences and needs.

It is important to recognize that a person's functional capacity does not always indicate the presence or degree of heart disease. Some individuals with severe heart disease are capable of vigorous exercise, while healthy but sedentary people may have the low levels of functional abilities that we usually associate with very limited cardiac cripples. Therefore, a training regimen should be tailored to the exercise capacity, as determined by the ability to perform continuous exercise. In healthy individuals, the heart is rarely the ultimate limiting factor; instead, it's the rest of the body—especially the legs —that need time to adjust to continuous vigorous exercise. Consequently, a thirty-five-year-old sedentary office worker, although free of heart disease, may perform at the same low exercise level as a fifty-year-old man who has had a severe heart attack but was in good physical shape beforehand. The expected rate of physical improvement for the two may be markedly different, but their starting point will be the same.

In order to minimize any inherent risks of exercise conditioning, all DUPAC participants are classified into three major groups:

1. Healthy people who have no indications of coronary disease.
2. People who may be at high risk for a heart attack.
3. People with established heart disease.

The actual exercise formats for each group are similar; indeed, all the groups exercise together at certain times. But the amounts of medical supervision for the heart patients and for the high-risk groups differ significantly. A physician is part of the exercise supervision team whenever new patients report to DUPAC. After a few months of exercise training, many patients find they no longer need to have a doctor present while working out; there are others, however, who may require lifelong supervision. Every patient is unique, and this is why it is so important that exercise conditioning be individualized for each person who has heart disease.

In addition to a physician, other members of the DUPAC exercise cardiac rehabilitation team include nurses, physician assistants, exercise physiologists, physical therapists, and physical educators. Heart patients are closely monitored during the initial stages of the program, with a staff therapist for every fifteen participants. People with severe disease may have one-to-one supervision during the first few weeks in order to maintain close watch for any potential symptoms of problems, and also to receive specific instructions. Should an emergency such as a heart attack or cardiac arrest occur, the emergency equipment is always close at hand. In DUPAC's eight years, there has been only one case of cardiac arrest while exercising, among the program's more than two thousand heart patients. This man was promptly resuscitated and treated, and was back in the program within a few days. On the average, only one serious cardiac event occurs for every ten thousand hours of exercise. "A heart patient is much more likely to die while asleep than during exercising," notes Paul Koisch.

It is also important to emphasize that even patients who are seriously limited by heart disease usually can benefit from exercise conditioning. Some have come to DUPAC with such severe disease that they could barely walk across the room. Sam B., a medical-school physician, was a case in point. He had suffered from progressively worsening heart disease for several years and had had several heart attacks, which had resulted in considerable damage. His heart's pumping ability was severely limited; he had advanced congestive heart failure and heart rhythm disturbances. He was on fourteen heart drugs, and even the least effort resulted in chest pain and shortness of breath. Within six weeks, he was able to walk around the Duke track and resume work on a medical textbook that he was editing. "We were unable to cure his heart disease," one of the DUPAC physicians explained, "but we were able to maximize even the very limited capacity that remained." Sam put it another way: "I came here fully expecting to die; instead, I learned how to live."

THE EXERCISE PRESCRIPTION

The basic components of the DUPAC exercise prescription are *intensity, frequency,* and *duration.* The optimal intensity of exercise is a rate sufficient to push the heart rate into the training range that has been determined by the exercise test. For healthy individuals who have not undergone an exercise test, the target training range can be estimated by taking into consideration normal resting heart rate, approximate maximum rate, and age.

Initially, there may be no urgency to push to the training range. Early on, the exercise routines emphasize volume and variety, not intensity. Just getting active is a good start: all joints, all muscles, all directions. For heart patients, particularly those on medication, the intensity and frequency become more important, months into the training program. It may take this long for the drug regimens to be adjusted, the joints and muscles to become accustomed to activity, and the elements of fear and uncertainty to be controlled.

The exercise sessions should be frequent enough to provide the desired conditioning effect. For DUPAC participants, this is five times a week. (Some other programs call for three or four sessions a week. This is the absolute minimum; five is highly preferred.)

Duration of exercise for heart patients at the DUPAC center ranges from forty minutes to two hours a day, depending on the individual's available time and the extent of the disease. If the allowable exercise intensity (training range) is very low, the longer sessions, involving a variety of exercises, may be best. For example, the patient may work out on the exercise bicycles for ten minutes at a fairly low work load, then participate in ten minutes of warm-up exercises, then walk at a moderate pace for thirty minutes, followed by ten minutes of cool-down exercises. Water walking in a special exercise pool may be added to the routine, to provide an additional half hour of exercise (or it may substitute for the track walking in people who have orthopedic problems). In contrast, a well-conditioned individual may need only forty minutes of more vigorous exercise to achieve the desired physiological effect. Everyone is unique, and will proceed at his or her own pace. But all participants have a common goal: to structure an exercise program that is efficient, fun, and safe, and that can be carried out in a home setting the year around.

START WITH WALKING

Walking is the single most useful exercise in the entire DUPAC cardiac exercise rehabilitation program. The ability to walk enables even the most seriously limited heart patient to regain a normal life. Almost any daily task is difficult, if not impossible, if your ability to walk is seriously hampered. Many people forget that walking is exercise, and it can be very vigorous exercise at that.

There are several reasons why the DUPAC exercise program revolves around walking. By walking, you can exercise the major muscle groups. For "reborn exercisers," the orthopedic considerations are paramount, especially for the older person. More would-be exercisers are sidelined by injuries to their joints, tendons, and muscles than heart considerations. The risk of trauma to the joints, bones, and muscles is an important element in designing an exercise program. No one is immune from athletic injury—even the world's finest runners suffer periodic breakdowns. The point at which an individual can be injured while walking or jogging may be surprisingly low. Good advice from the American Jogging Association: "Start slow and then slow down!" Remember, you have the rest of your life to attain fitness, to exercise in your training range, and to develop the stamina needed to enjoy life to the fullest.

Another important advantage of walking as a conditioning exercise is that, aside from appropriate footwear, you do not need any special equipment or facilities. DUPAC uses the Wallace Wade Football Stadium track, but any smooth, reasonably level, and safe walking area is suitable. A park, neighborhood sidewalks, shopping-mall lot, local schoolyard or athletic track, quiet country road or lane—all are possible walk areas.

Walking begins with adequate footwear. Years of sedentary living and, particularly among women, inappropriate shoes, may render your feet less than perfect for any increased use. But there is now such a variety of athletic footwear that almost everyone can be fitted with comfortable and appropriate walking and running shoes.

In selecting appropriate footwear, do not try to economize; good preventive orthopedics begins with good shoes. It's far better to scrimp on the unessentials—sweat suits, stopwatch, pulse meter, pedometer, Walkman radio, and all the other gear so many people embarking on an exercise program seem to splurge on—and instead buy a really good pair of shoes that are right for your feet and your needs. Prices vary, but you should expect to spend in the range of fifty dollars or more. Cheaper running/jogging shoes will not give you the service and support you need. By the same token, you do not need the top-of-the-line running shoes that can cost more than a hundred dollars. DUPAC patients are advised to go to a store that specializes in athletic footwear and to tell the salesperson what they will be using the shoes for. Many people think that any old pair of tennis shoes or inexpensive running shoes will do. Not so. Remember, too, that the newer walking/ jogging shoes are made of nylon or other synthetic fibers and will not "break in." So if they are uncomfortable in the store, don't buy them—they won't become any more comfortable with wear.

Initially, the intensity of the exercise training is not important. It's the act of making a definite commitment to exercise conditioning and the enjoyment of the activity that are important. The track segment of a DUPAC exercise session, for example, lasts thirty minutes. Patients shuffle, walk, jog, or wog (a combination of walking and jogging) as far as possible within their individualized exercise prescription. Some are able to jog the entire time; others may cover only a few hundred yards at a very slow pace. But, given time and perseverance, most can accomplish definite improvement.

Arthur P. is a typical case in point. He enrolled in DUPAC after a serious heart attack that had left considerable damage. At first, he could walk only four 100-yard intervals, with three minutes of rest between segments during the thirty-minute track session. It was little wonder, given his poor physical condition, that Mr. P.'s family physician had been dubious about the value of exercise conditioning for him. But after three months, Mr. P. was able to walk four complete laps, or one mile, in thirty minutes—a twelve-fold increase in exercise capacity. Although this is still a low level of exercise tolerance, he was then able to enjoy going to a shopping mall with his wife and a leisurely Sunday-afternoon stroll with his grandchildren. And he didn't stop there; over the next few months he continued to show improvement until he could walk seven laps (one and three quarters miles) in thirty minutes, and even jog a few steps in each lap, more for the novelty than athletic ambition. "Sure I jog," he says; "just don't ask how far!"

Once a DUPAC heart patient is able to establish a five-day-per-week walking regimen, the medical staff carefully evaluates his or her progress. Can the patient check his or her own pulse? Can the prescribed training range be reached? Are there any orthopedic considerations or worrisome symptoms? Are the more immediate medical needs being addressed adequately? Is it time to push for a faster pace, more laps, a higher heart rate? Generally, determined individuals of normal body weight and a healthy cardiovascular system make rapid gains in exercise capacity during the first few weeks or months. Heart disease, orthopedic problems, and obesity slow the training process, but even so, weekly improvement can be expected for most patients, especially after a weekend of rest and muscular rejuvenation—an important part of avoiding excessive fatigue and injury. There are, however, some patients that will take several weeks or months to show functional improvement. Still, almost everyone can benefit from some form of exercise rehabilitation.

JOGGING

The cadence of jogging is not significantly faster than brisk walking. But it is the up-and-down motion—indeed, the total body becomes airborne during the stride—that makes jogging a demanding cardiovascular exercise. The up-and-down motion is also the likely cause of the numerous joint, tendon, and muscle injuries experienced by so many joggers and runners. A few of the frequently seen injuries include:

- Frontal-compartment syndrome, or shin splints. The muscles along the fronts of the legs are overused and become swollen and painful.
- Achilles tendinitis. The tendon of the heel becomes inflamed, from either overuse or trauma, and painful.
- Lateral-collateral runner's knee. Overuse of the ligaments of the knee causes a painful form of bursitis (inflammation of the bursa, the fluid-filled sac that facilitates joint movement).
- Chondromalacia patellae, another form of bursitis, involving the kneecap.
- Plantar fasciitis, an inflammation of the sole of the foot.

These are but a few of the many orthopedic injuries experienced by runners and joggers. Jogging also can exacerbate existing joint problems such as osteoarthritis of the knees, hips, and ankles; and rheumatoid arthritis. Patients with these problems may need to concentrate on other forms of exercise.

Orthopedic injuries are usually a result of a structural imbalance of the limbs, and very often, one that is correctable. Unfortunately, one is often injured before the structural imbalance is diagnosed and corrected. Since running injuries are self-induced due to imbalance or overuse, and can be temporarily disabling, extra caution is needed before beginning.

The risk is also minimized by a gradual buildup of muscle and joint strength. DUPAC has developed a fifteen-stage jogging progression guideline to help reduce the risk of injury. This stage is reached only after a patient is able to monitor his or her exercise program and has established a comfortable walking base and it is time to strive for the aerobic training range. If the heart rate during walking is below the low end of the training range, the patient is instructed to speed up. This may involve more continuous walking with less resting until the full thirty-minute session is continuous exercise (water stops and pulse checks excepted). If it is above the high end of the training range, he or she is told to slow down.

Although many people, particularly heart patients, tend to measure their progress in terms of whether or not and how far they can jog, it should be emphasized that excellent exercise conditioning can be achieved by walking alone. In fact, walking is an Olympic track event, with some of the world's finest athletes competing. These race walkers can walk at 90 percent of their aerobic capacity for hours with heart rates of 160 or even higher. So why should a middle-aged DUPACer have difficulty walking fast enough to reach his or her exercise training range? In a word, technique. Why try to race walk, they may ask, when jogging will achieve the same heart rate and not look quite so difficult or strange?

In incorporating jogging into their walking regimens, DUPAC patients remain at each of the fifteen stages for at least one week. The hope is that if overuse injuries become a problem, they will be minor and walking can still be used as the cardiovascular stimulus. Patients are encouraged to take a very short stride, with a light, silent flat-footed touchdown. This may not be the way marathoner Bill Rodgers runs, but in the beginning, it minimizes the chance of injury. Advanced jogging techniques are appropriate only after two continuous miles of jogging can easily be achieved in under twenty minutes. Even patients who can easily achieve this goal rarely pursue advanced running styles, although there are those notable exceptions of formerly sedentary people who, after a heart attack, become so involved in running that they become marathoners. So long as one can establish a training routine that works and is beneficial and injury free, it seems pointless to change for the sake of change. Besides, change can create problems; very often, simply changing stride, speed, or even shoe brands can cause injury. In the words of Paul Koisch, "Go with what works best for you."

THE REST OF THE BODY

Although walking is the basic conditioning exercise used in the DUPAC training program, several other forms of physical activity are taught concomitantly. Stimulating the cardiovascular system may be the major goal, but it is important to realize that the heart is not the only body organ that benefits from exercise. Total fitness is achieved only by appropriate attention to all organ systems; thus the DUPAC approach includes the total body, and not just the cardiovascular system.

There are three major categories of exercise:

1. The repetitive, continuous dynamic muscle exercise, such as walking, that promotes aerobic training.

2. The stretching and joint-manipulation exercise, which often proceeds from or follows the more vigorous forms of exercise.

3. The exercises that promote strength and muscle mass. These include the muscle-leading exercises, which may be static (isometric) or dynamic (for example, Nautilus), which encourage the formation of lactic acid—a metabolic by-product of fatigued muscles—and short-term fatigue.

Some forms of exercise combine all three types. Also, the same exercise may have differing effects in various people. For example, Gerald S. can ride a stationary exercise bicycle (ergometer) at a work load of 300 kpm (kiloponds per minute) for twenty minutes, achieving category 1 exercise. In contrast, Sam B. can ride the same ergometer at the 300-kpm load for only two minutes before becoming short of breath and having his leg muscles become so tight or cramped that he can no longer turn the pedals. For Sam, this is category-3 exercise.

In general, heart patients should avoid category-3 exercise, especially if the upper-body muscle groups are involved or if the activity involves downward straining (e.g., weight lifting), resulting in a buildup of lung pressure by attempting to exhale against a closed glottis (the Valsalva maneuver). A buildup of lactic acid also should be avoided by heart patients if possible. Both the Valsalva maneuver and a buildup of lactic acid can increase the possibility of cardiac arrhythmia.

From a practical standpoint, some people must begin an exercise program by developing muscle strength before they can undertake endurance activities. The simple act of lifting the leg to take a step forward may be an arduous task for a heart-attack or surgery patient that has been in bed for several weeks. If the DUPAC rehabilitation team encounters this in a patient, the first step will be to design an exercise program that will develop muscle strength. If properly prescribed, even muscle-building exercises can be performed with a minimum of risk. Take the case of John L., for example. He had undergone a very complicated hospital course following his near-fatal heart attack. He could not walk on the treadmill for more than two minutes at a speed of 1.5 miles per hour before his legs became too tired to go on. His very low functional capacity required special consideration. A bicycle ergometer was selected as his initial training mode, and a program of no-load pedaling at a frequency of twenty-five pedal cycles per minute for two minutes was prescribed. The pedaling would be repeated after a brief rest interval. After ten days, John was able to repeat the work/rest cycle five times in thirty minutes. Considering the low work load—the weight of his own legs—he was not expending much energy, but it was his reasonable limit. After another ten days, John was able to combine a few yards of walking with the bike riding. Because of his fragile condition and symptoms of muscle fatigue, John required close medical supervision throughout his exercise session. Despite the low energy expenditure involved, it was an important beginning in John's rehabilitation process.

As illustrated by the case of John L., the bicycle ergometer is a very useful tool in early-stage cardiac rehabilitation. DUPAC prescribes the bicycle ergometer for all patients who have no orthopedic contraindications. The rationale is threefold:

1. It is easier to monitor patients on stationary bikes than it is when they are scattered on an exercise field.
2. It is possible to work out on a bicycle ergometer at any time of the year, something you cannot say for outdoor exercise.
3. It helps exercise the upper leg muscles more than walking can. This is important because well-conditioned quadriceps muscles help stabilize the knee and align the leg bones for optimal function.

The DUPAC daily exercise program begins with a stint of bicycle ergometry that is individually tailored to develop muscle tone. The bike session precedes the track workout and is a major portion of the early treatment phase. Eventually, many patients eliminate the ergometry in favor of stair climbing, Nautilus training, or walking/jogging. Others use ergometry as their major aerobic activity, and deemphasize walking and jogging. In this regard, the choice is largely one of individual preference. The bicycle ergometer can be adjusted to provide aerobic training by increasing the rate and load. At DUPAC, a typical cycling session may be less than ten minutes but at a rate of fifty revolutions per minute and a work load demanding enough to be challenging. It should be noted that most patients cannot work out in the training range until they have had several weeks of conditioning; disuse of the leg muscles has rendered the average American a rather poor cyclist.

STRETCHING

Stretching and joint manipulation are part of any well-rounded exercise program. DUPAC employs its stretching exercises as part of a choreographed warm-up routine before the track workout. The routine, called the DUPAC Daily Dozen, embodies muscle toning, joint manipulation, and stretching, in a complex progression of movement. At first, the exercises may be difficult to follow, but then, not everyone can foxtrot or boogie the first time he or she tries. Gradually, the movements become second nature and blend into a rhythmic prelude to the track work. The rate is expected to increase gradually throughout the course of the Daily Dozen, as the joints and muscles are called into action.

Adequate stretching is helpful in the prevention of muscle injury. Stretching is perhaps more critical for football players and other athletes who participate in "burst" sports that require short periods of very intensive physical activity. And as in anything, too much can be just as bad as too little; overstretching is a possibility, especially for older people. The important thing is to move, at first slowly and methodically, and then to increase the range and speed. Remember, no exercise, especially stretching movements, are performed quickly or in jerks. All movement should flow. The actual stretches are comfortable exercises with a minimal chance of overload, and when done in the sequence shown here (see pages 70–75), they are an ideal prelude to vigorous activity.

COOL-DOWN EXERCISES

Cool-down, or recovery, exercises are performed after the track (vigorous) routine and are designed to help the muscles readjust to the resting state. They also involve stretching movements, and thus provide a second opportunity to keep muscles limber. Tight, and even sore, muscles are often the consequence of undertaking an exercise program after years of sedentary living. The cool-down provides a transition to the resting state.

In essence, the cool-down routine is similar to the warm-up session, except the sequence is in reverse and muscle-relaxation exercises are added to help promote the feeling of well-being that exercise induces.

For heart patients, the cool-down session has added significance. Clinical studies suggest that it is during the after-exercise period that a person is most vulnerable to a heart attack or serious rhythm disturbance. The exercise stress test helps identify those patients who are at high risk for circumstances that may lead to a cardiac event, for example susceptibility to postexercise ischemia or abnormal heart rhythms. It should be emphasized that such problems are rare and the risk is small; even so, after-exercise precautions should be taken with as much diligence as the preparation phase. An added caution for heart patients: You should avoid a hot shower or sauna after exercise, because this puts an extra strain on the cardiovascular system. You also should make sure that you consume enough fluid to replace sweat loss.

WATER EXERCISE

Hydro-, or water, therapy has become an important part of the DUPAC program. The buoyant force of water can significantly reduce the stress on joints, particularly the knees and hips, that is inherent in walking. The DUPAC hydrotherapy pool is shallow—only forty-two inches deep—and has a flat bottom, rather than the tapered design found in most pools. It is intended more for water walking than for swimming. Although swimming is an excellent conditioning exercise, it is difficult to prescribe, because of the skill it requires and also the various physiological consequences of submergence. In contrast, water walking trains the same muscle groups used in walking on land but allows for a greater number of repetitions or steps before fatigue or orthopedic problems intervene.

These DUPAC patients perform water-walking exercise for thirty minutes, just as those who use the track. Periodic pulse checks are made, and the distance walked is expected to increase over several weeks of training.

There are some heart patients for whom water walking is not recommended; for example, people with borderline congestive heart failure are excluded from water walking. The same is true of extremely high-risk patients and those who have recently had heart surgery or a heart attack. The likelihood of a truly life-threatening emergency is rare, but a dizzy spell on the track is an example of a relatively minor event that could be much more serious should it occur in the water. DUPAC, of course, is prepared to handle emergencies, both on land and in the water.

In addition to water walking, DUPAC has devised a pool exercise regimen that is similar to aerobic dancing. This is particularly helpful in meeting the needs of older patients in total body conditioning. The exercises are designed to provide an aerobic workout for most individuals and involve repetitive jumps, swings, and movements that would be too strenuous for a land-based exercise program but that can be performed in water. In fact, with a few minor modifications in cadence, the water exercises can be used to challenge even the very fit. The obvious disadvantage to water exercise is the need for a special facility. Many people might not have access to an appropriate pool in their hometown setting.

WEIGHT LIFTING

The ability to lift weights is very important to many heart-attack patients, or even healthy formerly sedentary people, who are anxious to fully renew their physical abilities. Of course, there are also people who must be able to lift a certain amount of weight to return to their jobs. Thus, weight lifting is incorporated into the DUPAC rehabilitation program. Specific types of exercise equipment used in weight training include:

- Schwinn Airdyne ergometer, which allows for a continuous arm workout and involves a variety of muscles, depending upon the way it is used.
- Nautilus and Universal mechanical weight-training devices.
- One-hand dumbbells.

The type of weight-lifting equipment that will be used depends upon a number of factors, including the extent of heart disease and the preference of the individual. The Airdyne is the easiest equipment to master, and it uses most of the upper body. Dumbbells may be the best choice for people who must regain the ability to use a certain upper body movement in their jobs. Dumbbells are also inexpensive and easy to use at home. The dumbbells used at DUPAC range from two to ten pounds, in two-pound increments. Before beginning to work out with dumbbells, however, a heart patient should be instructed in motions that are most appropriate for him or her by a physician or exercise physiologist.

Nautilus and Universal equipment are used to meet specific needs and desires. After a year of therapy, some patients progress to a standard program of weight training, while others may still be limited to rather low-level activities. Like all forms of upper-body muscle conditioning, Nautilus and Universal workouts supplement the basic aerobic components of DUPAC and are used only after considerable levels of aerobic exercise are achieved. In general, heart patients would be advised to follow a similar progression of building strength and aerobic capacity by walking before enrolling in a Nautilus or Universal program. In fact, many rehabilitation programs would not even consider weight conditioning for heart patients, and with good reason. Weight lifting greatly increases the back pressure on the heart. Thus, cardiac patients must lift weights differently from healthy athletes. The object is to work only one muscle group at a time, and *never* to strain. Comfortable fatigue in the muscle group being exercised is permissible; total fatigue is not. Even healthy individuals should undertake weight training under expert supervision, and this is all the more true for heart patients. Very often, the role of the therapist becomes one of urging the heart patient to slow down, because of excessive exertion. Therefore, the only DUPAC patients who weight train are those who have:

- demonstrated an ability to monitor their own exercise, for example those who regularly check their own heart rates;
- achieved significant levels of aerobic conditioning;
- stayed within their prescribed exercise limits;
- attended regular exercise classes; and
- received appropriate medical clearance.

DUPAC has developed a very simple floor exercise routine that fills the need for a total body conditioning routine that is appropriate for most heart patients. The exercises, referred to as the Basic Six, are muscle-toning movements, with each exercise providing a muscle contraction phase and a non-weight-bearing, relaxation phase. You inhale during the contraction phase and exhale during relaxation. The number of times each exercise is repeated depends upon physical condition. Generally, the Basic Six are performed in rapid succession, with the total routine taking less than ten minutes. Three to five exercise sessions per week are recommended. (The Basic Six are illustrated on pages 76–79.)

SUMMING UP

Exercise conditioning is the cornerstone of the DUPAC approach to cardiovascular rehabilitation. By determining just how much functional capacity the heart has, it is possible to design an exercise program that will maximize this capability. Even heart patients who are seriously limited by their disease can make full use of remaining heart function and, in many instances, again lead normal lives. The benefits are worth the effort: the entire body will gain in strength, and you will achieve a renewed sense of well-being. It is a mistake to think that only heart patients benefit from exercise conditioning; a healthy but sedentary person can reap the same rewards, and perhaps even prevent or delay a heart attack.

THE DUPAC DAILY DOZEN

Warming Up

1. *Shoulder and Arm Circles:* 16 times
   Circle your shoulders backward. Gradually increase the size of the rotation to include your arms. Bend your knees every time your arms go around.

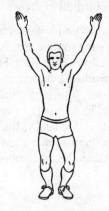

2. *Touchdowns:* 6 times
   Bend down—touch the floor (1, 2) (Bend your knees, not your back) and —stretch up (3, 4).

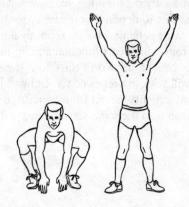

3. *Side Bends:* 3 times each side
   With your arms above your head, bend to the left and stretch (1) (no bouncing)—bend to the right (2).

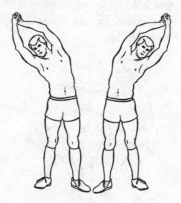

4. *Side Twists:* 6 times each side
   Swing your arms from side to side and twist.

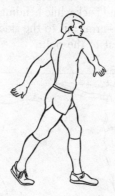

5. *Hamstring Stretch:*
   Assume a slight knee-bent position, with your heels flat and toes pointed straight ahead, for fifteen seconds. Stand up and bend forward with your knees slightly bent and hold on to your ankles with your hands. Stretch the hamstrings for ten seconds. Do not bounce. Repeat. Bend your knees more when you rise or stand up.

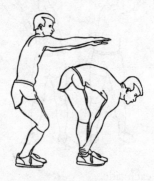

6. *Down-and-Out Swing:* 6 times each side
   Swing your arms down and back while bending your knees (1). Swing your arms up and stretch (2)—arms out to the sides, left leg out to the left—and bounce (3, 4). Repeat to the right.

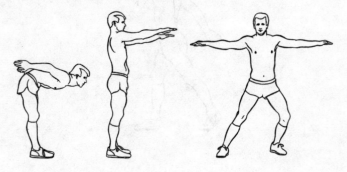

7. *Inner-Thigh Stretch:*
   Stand with your legs apart, your left knee bent and your body weight on your left leg. Put both hands on your left knee as support. Toes should point forward. Gradually press your right leg down toward the ground. Tense the inner thigh muscle. Hold for ten seconds. Relax the muscle two to three seconds and then stretch the inner thigh again by bending your left knee a little more for ten more seconds. Repeat for the left leg.

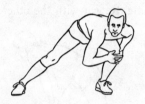

8. *Side Swing:* 4 times each side
   Stand with your legs apart and both arms up to the right. Swing both arms down to the floor while bending your knees (1) and up to the left side while stretching and reaching (2). Repeat, swinging back to the right side.

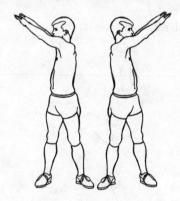

9. *Calf Stretch:*

Stand with your legs apart, one foot in front of the other, the knee slightly bent, and both hands on the bent knee as support. The other leg should be straight, with the toes pointed forward and the heel on the floor. Press the heel down to the floor—tense the calf muscle for ten seconds. Relax the muscle for two to three seconds and then stretch the calf muscle for ten seconds by slowly moving your hips forward. Be sure to keep the heel on the floor all the time. Repeat with the other leg.

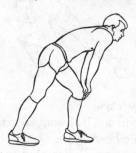

10. *Kicks:* 5 times each leg

Kicks with clap above head.

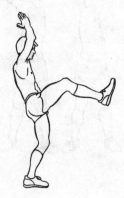

11. *Cross-Country Skiing:* 16 times
    Swing your arms, one forward and one back, while moving up and down with your knees.

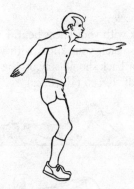

12. *Down, Up, and Around Swing:* 8 times
    Swing your arms down and back while bending your knees (1). Swing your arms up while stretching your knees (2). Swing your arms around while bending your knees (3).

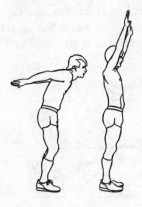

THE BASIC SIX FOR ALL-AROUND FITNESS

1. *Modified Sit-Ups:*

   For the abdominal muscles:

   Lie down on your back with your knees bent. Raise your shoulders (about 30 degrees) and try to reach your knees with your fingertips. The lower (lumbar) region of your back should stay on the ground at all times. Hold for eight to ten seconds. Relax. (10 times)

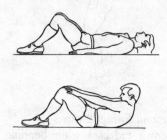

   Variations:

   A. Try to reach your left knee and then your right knee.
   B. Try the exercise with your arms crossed on your chest.
   C. Try the exercise with your hands behind your head.
   D. Try the exercise with your arms above your head.

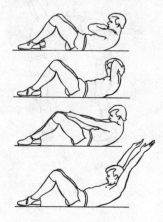

2. *Back-Ups:*
   For your arm, thigh, leg, and back muscles:
   Sit down on the floor with your hands as support behind you. Lift up your
   hips (1), down again (2). Bend forward and touch your toes with your
   knees slightly bent (3) and back again (4). (10 times)

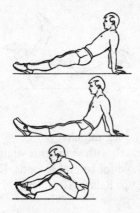

3. *Upper Back:*
   For your upper-back and shoulder muscles:
   Lie down on your stomach. Pull your elbows back toward the middle of
   your spine. Keep your neck straight and look at the floor. Hold for eight to
   ten seconds. Relax. (10 times)

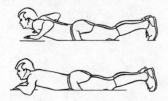

4. *Fanny Exercise:*
   For your buttocks:
   Lie down on your stomach with your knees bent. Lift up your left knee and hold for several seconds. Down and relax. Lift your right knee up. Relax. (10 times or 5 with each knee)

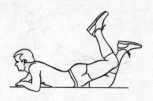

5. *Back Exercise:*
   For your back, arm, and leg muscles:
   Lie down on your stomach with your arms straight ahead. Lift your right arm and left leg and hold for several seconds. Down and relax. Lift your left arm and right leg up. Relax. (10 times or 5 with each side)

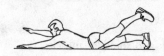

6. *Push-Ups:*

For your arm muscles:
Push-up or modified push-up. Down and relax. Clap your hands between push-ups. (10 times)

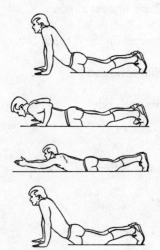

COOLING DOWN

Exercises 1 through 9 are the same as those included in the warm-up; exercises 10 through 12 are illustrated here.

1. Down, Up, and Around Swing: 8 times

2. Cross-Country Skiing: 16 times

3. Side Swing: 4 times each side

4. Hamstring Stretch

5. Down-and-Out Swing: 6 times

6. Inner-Thigh Stretch

7. Side Twists: 5 times each side

8. Calf Stretch

9. Side Bends: 3 times each side

10. Wake-Up Stretch: 3 times

Bend forward with knees bent. Relax head, arms, and shoulders. Gradually uncurl and stretch both arms above your head while inhaling. Exhale, relax, and repeat.

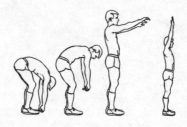

11. Arm Relaxer: 3 times

Lift both arms slowly halfway up while inhaling. Drop arms down while exhaling.

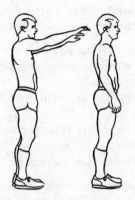

12. Shoulder Relaxer: 4 times

Tense and lift both shoulders while inhaling. Drop shoulders and relax while exhaling.

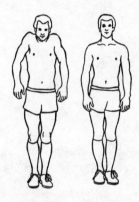

Finish with one large shoulder and arm circle.

DUPAC'S EXERCISE PRESCRIPTION

To properly train the heart muscle, several variables need to be specified. The basics of exercise prescription are as follows:

A. Type of exercise—walking, jogging, swimming, cycling, or any sustained rhythmic activity of enough intensity to elevate the heart rate into the "training range."

B. Duration—the length of time your heart should operate in the training range.

C. Frequency—the number of bouts per week needed to promote and maintain cardiovascular fitness.

D. Intensity—reflected in the "training range."

The intensity should be custom tailored for you, based on the stress test. Duration and frequency are specified as minimums and are done for thirty minutes at least three times per week.

SUGGESTED PROGRESSIVE WALKING PROGRAM FOR CARDIAC PATIENTS: A

(As determined by results of exercise tolerance test; program is more strenuous than B)

Weeks	Distance (miles)	Time Goal (min.)	Freq./Wk.
1–2	1.0	20:00	5
3–4	1.0	17:30	5
5–6	1.0	15:00	5
7–8	1.5	23:00	5
9–10	1.5	22:30	5
11–12	2.0	31:00	5
13–14	2.0	30:00	5
15–16	1.5	21:30	5
17–18	1.5	21:00	5
19–20	2.0 and 2.5	28:45 36:00	3 2
21–22	2.0 and 2.5	28:30 35:45	3 2
23–24	2.5 and 3.0	35:30 43:15	4 1
25–26	2.5 and 3.0	35:15 43:15	3 2
27–28	2.5 and 3.0	35:00 42:30	3 2
29–30	3.0	42:00	5
31–32	4.0	55:00	3

MINIMAL REQUIREMENTS TO MAINTAIN FITNESS AFTER COMPLETION OF CONDITIONING PROGRAM A

Distance (miles)	Time Goal (min.)	Freq./Wk.
1.5 (twice a day)	18:00–21:44	5
or 2.0	24:00–28:59	8
or 3.0	36:00–43:29	5
or 4.0	48:00–57:59	3
or 5.0	72:30–99:59	4

SUGGESTED PROGRESSIVE WALKING PROGRAM
FOR CARDIAC PATIENTS: B

(As determined by results of exercise tolerance test;
program is more gradual than A)

Weeks	Distance (miles)	Time Goal (min.)	Freq./Wk.
1–2	1.0	24:00	5
3–4	1.0	20:00	5
5–6	1.0	18:00	5
7–8	1.0	16:00	5
9–10	1.5	25:00	5
11–12	1.5	24:00	5
13–14	2.0	33:00	5
15–16	2.0	32:00	5
17–18	1.5	23:00	2
	and		
	2.5	40:00	3
19–20	1.5	22:30	2
	and		
	3.0	47:00	3
21–22	2.5	38:00	2
	and		
	3.5	54:00	3
23–24	2.5	36:00	3
	and		
	3.0	44:00	2
25–26	3.0	43:15	3
	and		
	4.0	61:00	2
27–28	3.0	43:15	3
	and		
	4.0	60:00	2
29–30	3.0	43:00	5
31–32	4.0	57:45	3

MINIMAL REQUIREMENTS TO MAINTAIN FITNESS AFTER
COMPLETION OF CONDITIONING PROGRAM B

Distance (miles)	Time Goal (min.)	Freq./Wk.
1.5 (twice a day)	18:00–21:44	5
or 2.0	24:00–28:59	8
or 3.0	36:00–43:29	5
or 4.0	48:00–57:59	3
or 4.0	58:00–79:59	4
or 5.0	72:30–99:59	3

DUPAC'S RULES FOR JOGGING

Orthopedic Injury—Enemy Number One

A. Up to 90 percent of running injuries are avoidable if the exercise is followed systematically and with regularity. If any area of the body, such as the knees, shins, or hips, are sore, allow at least one week of pain-free walking before attempting to jog.

B. Purchase good-quality running shoes to help prevent injuries.

C. Jogging injuries are self-imposed. Jogging through leg pain may have serious consequences. If the pain will not go away after a week's rest, see a doctor.

D. Brisk walking, bicycling, or swimming can be every bit as "aerobic" as jogging. Do the form of exercise that is best suited for you!

Coping with the Urge to Do Too Much

A. "Train, don't strain."

B. Jog only hard enough to be in your training heart-rate range.

C. Don't jog so hard that you can't carry on a conversation with the person next to you.

D. Smile when you jog, so others will think you are having fun.

E. "Sprinting at the end of a training run is strictly bush-league." (Frank Shorter)

F. Don't get too time-conscious. Enjoy the exercise and use the training schedules only as a rough guide. Progress at your own rate!

Jogging in Hot Weather

A. Drink water before, after, and during jogging.

B. Expose as much skin as possible to the air during hot weather.

C. Check your heart rate. Hot weather by itself will increase the cardiac demand.

D. Do not try to jog in a rubber suit.

E. Avoid salt tablets in favor of lots of water.

F. The two hundred to three hundred calories burned during an exercise session will not cause several pounds of weight loss, but an excessive loss of body fluid might. Replace any weight loss during jogging with an equivalent weight in fluids.

Eating

A. A well-balanced diet is essential to athletic performance.

B. Strenuous exercise dulls the appetite. Plan meals after a running session to help with weight loss.

C. Obese individuals should not jog until weight loss is accomplished. Walking is the preferred exercise.

D. Eating before exercise can cause stomach cramping and reduced performance.

Jogging Techniques

A. The foot strikes should be *flat*-footed, with a light touchdown.

B. The stride length should be short to very short.

C. The foot recovery should be a shuffle, less than one inch off the ground.

D. A person jogging behind you should not be able to see the soles of your shoes.

E. The shoulder and neck muscles should be completely relaxed.

F. Advanced jogging/running techniques should be considered only after a firm mileage base of fifteen miles per week for three months.

Jogging Pace

A. Learning pace helps prevent fatigue and ensures the proper intensity of the exercise for maximum benefit.

B. Hundred-yard jog test: After measuring a hundred-yard course (a football field is a convenient place to learn pace), time yourself for the distance.

Beginning joggers should cover the distance in about forty seconds or more. Experienced joggers should jog a hundred yards in about twenty-seven seconds. Forty-one seconds is equal to twelve minutes per mile; thirty-five seconds is equal to ten minutes per mile; twenty-seven seconds is equal to eight minutes per mile.

Goals for Workouts

   A. Workouts should last at least thirty minutes.

   B. The distance covered should be at least two miles.

   C. Maintain your own pace and increase the speed only if you are injury free and reasonably comfortable, and then decrease your time per mile only by a modest amount, about ten to twenty seconds per mile.

   D. Walkers will need to commit more time to training in order to obtain equivalent aerobic benefit.

   E. Three workouts per week is a minimum requirement for physical fitness. Although the walking and jogging progressions are designed for a three-day-per-week commitment, any extra time invested will help speed up the conditioning process. Allow at least one day per week of rest.

   F. If illness or work causes interruptions in the training schedule, reduce the workout intensity to allow the body to readjust. Most serious problems occur in "reborn athletes" after a period of abstinence.

   G. Allow an additional few minutes for warm-up and cool-down with each exercise session.

Taking Your Heart Rate

   A. Find a place on your body where you can feel your pulse. Try the neck (carotid) artery (one side only).

   B. Count your pulse for ten seconds. For the beats per minute, multiply by six.

   C. Practice enough so you can teach others to do it.

Other Exercises
to Supplement a Jogging Program

A. Stair climbing: Jogging develops the lower legs but does little for the quadriceps (thigh) muscles. Seven to ten flights of stairs every other day or so will help tone the quads. Heart-rate rules apply for stair climbing, too. Do not exceed your training range.

B. DUPAC Basic Six.

DUPAC'S GUIDELINES FOR HOME
EXERCISE PROGRAMS

In establishing a practical home exercise program, there are several factors that must be considered:

1. You must make it a regular part of your schedule. Many people find it easiest to exercise first thing in the morning, before the activities of the day crowd in.

2. It is important that you exercise at least three nonconsecutive days each week during which times your heart rate accelerates to the prescribed level for thirty to forty minutes.

3. Is there a group of individuals in your community involved in similar cardiovascular exercise—a YMCA or church group? If so, you might investigate their program for your own purposes. It is usually easier to stick to an exercise program if there is someone else expecting you to exercise. Friends and fellow exercisers can also serve as an often needed source of support and encouragement.

4. Your exercise program does not need to require the purchase of any special equipment other than a pair of supportive and comfortable running shoes and a bathing suit. Adjust your routine to available facilities: a local high school or college track, a YMCA pool, or the sidewalk in your neighborhood.

5. Each exercise session should include a ten-to-fifteen-minute warm-up period that includes light calisthenics and gentle stretching (no bouncing or overstretching—if it is painful, you are overdoing it) involving both arms and legs as well as your trunk.

6. The main emphasis of a cardiovascular conditioning program is the aerobic phase, in which the heart rate is elevated into the prescribed training range continuously for thirty to forty minutes. This aerobic exercise can be attained via several activities such as walking/jogging, water walking/swimming, stationary bicycling, or stationary rowing. (Progressions for each are described later.) The intensity of this exercise (how fast the pace of walking or swimming, the resistance of bicycle and rowing ergometers) is modulated according to the level necessary for maintenance of the training heart rate.

7. Following this aerobic phase, it is important that you allow your body to "cool down" gradually afterward, letting your heart rate and any other physiological responses to exercise return to their resting levels.

8. Keep a daily record of your exercise. This need be only a simple chart with the date, distance covered, time of continuous exercise, maximum ten-

second pulse count, and any symptoms or comments you might want to add. This will show your progress over the ensuing weeks, for both your own satisfaction and your physician's information.

9. Do not exercise immediately following a meal; wait at least thirty minutes.

10. Be flexible. If you have had a physically exerting day at work or at home and you feel fatigued prior to exercise, adjust your exercise accordingly. If you are truly exerted, your heart rate will increase to your target with a lower level of exercise. That's fine! You don't need to feel compelled to match the previous session's level of exercise.

Special Tips for Hot-Weather Exercise:

1. Plan your exercise for the cooler parts of the day: early morning or after dinner.

2. Wear loose-fitting, light-weight clothing.

3. When exercising in high heat and/or humidity, your body is under greater cardiovascular stress. Therefore it is important that you check your heart rate frequently. You may need to adjust the intensity of your exercise to avoid going above your training heart rate.

4. The body's method of cooling itself in hot weather is to increase perspiration. This often results in dehydration if precautions are not taken to avoid heat stress. These include drinking plenty of water before, during, and after exercise (carry a bottle of water with you to the gym or track if a water fountain is not accessible).

Walk/Jog

1. Keep a daily record. Chart the date, distance covered, time of continuous walking, maximum ten-second pulse count, and any symptoms or comments you might want to add.

2. Warm-up (ten to fifteen minutes). This should include stretching for flexibility (slow holding stretch—should not feel painful), modified push-ups, and bent-knee sit-ups (knees down on floor, tuck chin to chest, and curl up so that shoulders are off the floor) to increase strength.

If you have a stationary bicycle or a rowing machine, you may use this as part of your warm-up.

3. Walk thirty to forty minutes continuously on three nonconsecutive days per week. Swing your arms and stride along at an even, rhythmic pace. This pace will be determined by your training heart-rate range.

Check your heart rate after three to five minutes of walking. If you are within your prescribed training range, maintain that pace. If you are below your training range, increase your pace to a brisker walk; if you are above your maximum, slow down a little. Check again after fifteen to twenty minutes, adjusting your pace to stay within your training range. Take a final pulse immediately upon finishing your thirty minutes of walking and/or jogging.

As you continue with your walking program, you will notice that you have to increase your pace to maintain your heart rate in your prescribed training range. This is a good sign of your improving level of conditioning.

You may reach a point where even your briskest walk doesn't increase your heart rate enough. At this time, if your doctor approves, you need to begin alternating short intervals of slow jogging with your brisk walk; or, if you can't jog for orthopedic or other reasons but have access to a football stadium or other facility with several flights of stairs, walk ten minutes, then climb the stadium stairs halfway. Come down and repeat until you have exercised for thirty to forty minutes. When this no longer serves to increase your heart rate into your training range, climb the entire stadium stairs, or six or seven flights, in the intervals between periods of walking.

4. If you develop any of the following symptoms during or after your walk, report to your physician:

   a. excessive fatigue
   b. any unusual joint, muscle, or ligament problem
   c. chest pain
   d. pain in the teeth, jaws, arms, or ear
   e. light-headedness, or dizziness
   f. nausea and/or vomiting
   g. headache
   h. shortness of breath
   i. sustained increase in heart rate after slowing
      down or resting
   j. irregularity of pulse

5. Cool down: a five-minute period of easy walking followed by gentle stretching exercises.

Aerobic Alternatives

Bicycle:

1. Warm-ups as for walking/jogging.

2. Five minutes of bicycle warm-up at an intensity that keeps your heart rate ten to twenty beats below your training range. Increase the intensity of breaking resistance to your prescribed kp (kiloponds or degree of resistance) level. Pedal at 50 rpm continuously for thirty to forty minutes, checking your heart rate as in walking/jogging.

Final two to three minutes, lower resistance to 0 kp for cool-down.

3. Cool-down stretching and calisthenics.

Swimming/Water Walking

1. Warm-ups on deck of pool as in walking/jogging.
2. Water exercises: five minutes to allow body to adjust to water temperature of pool.
3. Walk width of pool in the three-to-four-foot depth, keeping track of number of lengths walked.
4. Walk for thirty minutes using your heart training range as a guide to speed of walking.
5. Cool down.

DUPAC'S FIFTEEN-STAGE JOGGING PROGRAM

Very few people can undertake jogging without a progressive buildup of both stamina and muscular strength. If you have problems walking briskly for two or three miles, it would be folly to think you can take up jogging without even more problems. Jogging and running are particularly hard on weight-bearing joints: knees, ankles, and feet. If you have any orthopedic problems, such as arthritis, a bad back, joint problems, it may be wise to concentrate on other forms of aerobic exercise, such as walking or swimming. But if jogging is considered an appropriate form of exercise for you, here's a model progression program designed to minimize problems.

Stage	Distance jogged	Duration	Instructions
		Level One	
1	0 to 25 yards	30 minutes	Use a quarter-mile
2	25 yards	3–5 times a	track if possible;
3	50	week	jog the indicated
4	75		distance on each
5	100		lap; walk briskly
			when not jogging.
			Spend at least one
			week at each
			stage; longer if
			problems develop.
		Level Two	
6	1/2 lap	30 minutes	A trip around the
7	3/4 lap	3–5 times a	track is a lap; each
8	1 lap	week	quarter of that is
9	1 1/2 laps		110 yards. For
10	2 laps		each distance
			jogged, walk 110
			yards. Spend at
			least one week at
			each stage; cut
			back on jogging if
			problems develop.

Stage	Distance jogged	Duration	Instructions
		Level Three	
11	3 laps	30 minutes	Again, intersperse
12	4 laps	3–5 times a	the segments
13	5 laps	week	jogged with
14	6 laps		walking 110 yards,
15	Continuous jogging		until you reach
			stage 15.

Diet and the Heart

CASE HISTORY

Bob N. lived to eat. The day would start with a hearty southern breakfast: six or seven strips of bacon, two eggs fried in the bacon grease, grits flavored with bacon fat and syrup, two or three slices of toast slathered with butter and jam, two or three cups of coffee with sugar and cream. Midmorning, he would have three or four doughnuts and another cup of coffee. Midday would see him sit down to a full dinner; typically two or three pork chops or a thick slice of southern ham, fried potatoes, beans cooked with fatback, several rolls or slices of bread with jam and butter, a couple of slices of pie, and again two or three cups of coffee. The supper menu would be similar, but with larger portions and accompanied by two or three bottles of beer. Before going to bed, he would raid the refrigerator and make a couple of sandwiches and have another piece of pie and a couple of glasses of whole milk. Although only forty-three years old, he looked much older and weighed 260 pounds. He had high blood pressure and elevated cholesterol, and he smoked two packs of cigarettes a day.

Bob's job as a supervisor in charge of a maintenance crew involved a good deal of stress and more administrative work than physical labor. He seldom engaged in any physical activity away from his job—his main leisure-time pursuits were watching TV or napping or having a few beers with the fellows. Walking up stairs or other exertion left him feeling winded, but he attributed this to his weight. Except for being overweight, Bob considered himself to be in relatively good health.

Then, one day, he suffered a heart attack. It happened at work and he was rushed to the Duke Medical Center. He was in the hospital for two weeks and was then sent home to recuperate for another four months before returning to work. His doctor had told him he should quit smoking. He managed to stop the cigarettes, but he increased the number of cigars. He had also been given a strict weight-reduction diet that allowed twelve hundred calories a day and eliminated most of his favorite foods: bacon, ham, pie, fried potatoes, steak, donuts, butter, eggs, cream. . . . He was put on antihypertensive medication, which he took twice a day. He tried to stick to the diet, but after a few weeks he began to gradually slip back to his former eating habits, and the eighteen pounds he had lost in the hospital and during his early recuperation were quickly regained.

When Bob returned to work, he began to have angina. "I couldn't climb a flight of stairs or walk seventy-five feet without having to stop several times," he recalls. Finally, he returned to the Duke Medical Center, where he underwent cardiac catheterization and a complete medical workup. Although he had severe coronary-artery disease, he was not considered a good candidate for bypass surgery. Instead, his doctor recommended that he try DUPAC. "I knew I had to do something, and I was ready to try anything," he says. The day after he was released from his second hospital stay, he enrolled in the DUPAC as a medical patient.

"At first it was murder," he told us. "I couldn't make it around the track once. Even the warm-up exercises left me completely winded. I'd watch the others climb up all the stadium stairs at the end of a session and think, 'I'm never going to do that.' "

Both Bob and his wife, who was also markedly overweight, began to eat all their weekday meals at DUPAC. "The refrigerator was kept empty except for a few carrots, juice, and fruit. For the first time in my life, I stuck to a diet."

Gradually, his endurance began to increase. After four months, he said, "I still can't jog, but I can make it around the track four or five times." At the end of a session, he manages to climb the stadium stairs, even though he stops to rest a couple of times on the way. He has lost twenty-five pounds and has set a goal of twenty-five more.

"I no longer live to eat," he says, "even though I feel hungry all the time, and sometimes dream about ham and eggs." A typical breakfast is now orange juice and a bowl of oatmeal. Twice a week he will have an egg. "I probably shouldn't, but considering I used to eat more than a dozen eggs a week, cutting back to two is pretty good." His doctors agree.

Because of his high blood pressure, Bob has been instructed to cut back on salt—something that has been almost as hard as reducing his total food intake. But his wife is learning new ways of cooking and to use herbs instead of salt for flavoring. "At first, things just don't taste right without salt, but after a while your taste buds adjust. Now I actually prefer the taste of vegetables cooked without salt."

Bob is now able to perform most of his functions at work. "I probably never will be able to hustle around the way I used to," he says, "but I now know my limits. And I feel better than I have for years."

While the case of Bob N. is an extreme one, it illustrates the possible role of dietary excess in the development of heart disease and the important role of dietary modification in treating it. Although doctors have recognized the association between nutrition and certain diseases for centuries, it has been only in recent decades that heart disease has been linked to diet. The Framingham Heart Study, for example, has identified two nutrition-linked factors that increase our risk of heart attacks: high levels of blood cholesterol, which is associated with a diet high in saturated fats, and obesity, the result of chronic overeating. In addition, many experts believe that excessive salt consumption may be a factor in developing high blood pressure.

Americans enjoy an abundance of food unprecedented in human history. Modern agriculture and transportation make it possible to obtain food from every part of the world throughout the year. Walk into any supermarket and you are likely to find hams from Poland, spring lamb from New Zealand, exotic delicacies from the Orient, cheese from France and Italy, a dazzling array of fresh fruits and vegetables in any season, and, of course, foods from every part of the United States. What's more, our food prices are among the lowest of any nation. This abundance exists despite the fact that hunger remains a global problem. Indeed, it is ironic that overeating is now a major American health problem, at a time when most of the world's population does not get enough to eat. But not only do large numbers of Americans overeat, we also tend to consume a diet that is generally too high in fat, salt, and simple carbohydrate such as sugar, and too low in complex carbohydrate and fiber. Although an extreme case, the diet consumed by Bob, the DUPAC patient just described, represents an example of eating far too much and consuming large quantities of the wrong things.

THE ROLE OF CHOLESTEROL AND FATS

There are many misconceptions and considerable confusion about cholesterol and fats and their possible roles in the development of coronary disease. To clarify some of these misunderstandings, let's first define some of the basic terms used in discussing fats.

There are three basic types of fats: *Saturated* fats, so determined by their composition, are found mostly in animal products, such as butter, whole milk, and animal fat. *Unsaturated* fats, also determined by their composition, are found mostly in vegetable sources, particularly the liquid oils from corn, cottonseed, safflower, and sunflower and sesame seeds. Saturated fats tend to be hard or solid at room temperature; unsaturated fats are soft or liquid. *Monosaturated fats* fall between the saturated and the unsaturated fats and are often referred to as neutral fats, because they don't affect cholesterol levels. *Total fat* refers to all fat, regardless of whether it is saturated or unsaturated. All fats are higher in calories than proteins and carbohydrates: one gram of fat contains about nine calories, while one gram of protein or carbohydrate yields about four calories.

Cholesterol, although often mistakenly referred to as a fat, is actually a sterol lipid, a fatlike alcohol of high molecular weight. It is found only in products of animal origin, most notably the brain, nerves, liver, blood, and bile. Dietary sources include egg yolks, animal fats (particularly those in organ and red meats), and dairy products, such as cream and cheese. It is essential to maintain nerve function, cell structure, reproduction—in short, life itself. Although cholesterol is needed to maintain life, it is not necessary to consume any in the diet; the body is capable of manufacturing all that it needs. (The cholesterol produced by the body is known as endogenous cholesterol, while that consumed in food is called exogenous cholesterol.)

The possible link between high cholesterol and atherosclerosis was first documented in 1913 by a Russian pathologist, Nikolai Nikolaevich Anichkov, who showed that rabbits fed a high-cholesterol diet developed hardening of the arteries. Of course, humans are very different from rabbits, but further studies since then have repeatedly found that population groups that consume a diet high in cholesterol and saturated fats tend to have higher-than-normal levels of blood cholesterol. These people also have a high rate of heart attacks.

Although diet plays a major role in determining the level of cholesterol and other lipids that circulate in the blood, the story of how the body manufactures and uses cholesterol is more complicated than a simple matter of supply and demand. Since lipids are fatty substances and fats are not soluble in water (the major component of blood), they must be attached to another substance that is water soluble before they can be transported through the body. This substance is a protein molecule, which, when combined with the lipid, forms a molecule called a lipoprotein. These lipoproteins come in various sizes, and the amount of cholesterol and other fats they carry varies according to weight and size. The largest, the high-density lipoproteins, or HDL, have the highest proportion of protein, and recent studies have found HDL cholesterol seems to carry fat away from body cells and is therefore important in helping prevent the accumulation of cholesterol and other fats along the artery walls. In contrast, low-density lipoprotein, or LDL, contains the largest proportion of cholesterol of all the lipoproteins. The LDL molecule is lighter than the HDL, and it appears to carry cholesterol to the cells. Thus, a high level of LDL in the blood is considered instrumental in the development of atherosclerosis. There is still another lipoprotein, the very-low-density lipoprotein, or VLDL, and it carries the largest amount of triglycerides. It is important in the manufacture of other lipoproteins, but its role, if any, in atherosclerosis has not yet been defined.

It is clear, however, that while the level of total cholesterol is important, its composition in terms of lipoproteins is also important. The higher the ratio of HDL to LDL the better. A number of factors have been found to influence this ratio. Heredity is a major determinant: Some families tend to have high HDL levels, and studies have found that these people have a low incidence of heart attacks and live longer than average. In contrast, people with an inherited disorder known as familial hypercholesterolemia have extraordinarily high levels of LDL, and unless treated, usually die from heart disease at a very early age. Diabetics also have a high LDL/HDL ratio. A number of other factors also influence the LDL/HDL ratio. Women tend to have a higher level of HDL than men. People who engage in vigorous exercise, especially long-distance runners, enjoy high levels of HDL. Vegetarians also have high HDL. All of these groups tend to have a lower incidence of coronary disease, further documenting the desirability of having a high level of HDL cholesterol. In contrast, smokers tend to have a low level of HDL, and of course smokers also have a higher incidence of heart attacks.

What is considered an ideal cholesterol level? In general, the average cholesterol level is higher in the United States and other industrialized countries than in less-developed, agrarian societies. Most U.S. doctors consider a cholesterol level of 220 milligrams per deciliter (mg./dl.) to be normal, but this is high by world standards. The incidence of heart attacks in people whose cholesterol is 200 mg./dl. or less is relatively low, while it is very high in people with cholesterol levels of 300 mg./dl. or more. But there are exceptions to both, and there is no level at which the risk can be predicted with 100 percent accuracy. And as stressed earlier, the total cholesterol is not the whole story; the ratio of HDL to LDL is also an important determining factor. In addition, the possible role in heart disease of triglycerides (the most plentiful lipid in the diet and one that is also manufactured in the body) has not been defined.

In any event, most experts agree that Americans generally consume more fat than they should and recommend that the amount of dietary fat be reduced to 30–35 percent of the total calories. The average American now consumes more than 40 percent of his or her calories in the form of fats. These fats range from butter, margarine, and the various oils or shortening used in cooking to fats hidden in processed foods, cereals, baked goods, meats, cheese, eggs, and other foods. Although many Americans are making a conscious effort to lower their consumption of cholesterol, the average diet still contains about 500 milligrams per day—much more than the 300 milligrams recommended by the American Heart Association.

The best way to reduce cholesterol intake is to cut back on foods from animal sources, since cholesterol is found only in animal products. Egg yolks are one of the most concentrated dietary sources; high amounts also are found in liver, sweetbreads, kidneys, brains, and hearts. Fatty red meats, such as well-marbled steaks, tend to be high in cholesterol. Shrimp are also relatively high in cholesterol, although not as high as fatty red meats. Whole milk and foods made from whole milk or cream—for example, cheese and butter—also are high in cholesterol and saturated fat. In a prudent, low-cholesterol diet, all of these foods are eaten in great moderation, if at all.

While saturated fats tend to raise blood cholesterol, polyunsaturated fats appear to lower it. Good sources of these fats include oils made from corn, safflower, sunflower seeds, cottonseed, sesame seeds, and soybeans. Monosaturated fats, which do not alter blood cholesterol, are found in olive and peanut oils. Saturated vegetable fats include palm and coconut oils, which are widely used in baked goods, shortening, nondairy creamers, whipped toppings, and some margarines; they raise the body's production of cholesterol and should be avoided by anyone trying to lower cholesterol levels. In addition, normally unsaturated fats can be subjected to a chemical process, hydrogenation, to make them harder and thus more saturated. Solid vegetable shortenings and hard margarines contain hydrogenated oils and should be used sparingly.

Anyone interested in lowering fat consumption must learn to read nutritional labels on foods and, indeed, also learn to look for hidden fats in many prepared foods. In particular, look for key terms such as hardened or hydrogenated. This means that extra hydrogen has been added to the fat molecule and that the fat—which may have started out as polyunsaturated—is now at least partially saturated. Preferred margarines, for example, are those that list liquid oils as the first ingredient and have at least a two-to-one ratio of polyunsaturated to saturated fats. In general, the softer the margarine or spread at room temperature, the higher the amount of polyunsaturated oil. Nutritional labels also may list the milligrams of cholesterol per serving. Baked goods, cake and cookie mixes, and prepackaged convenience foods tend to be high in saturated fats. Menus and recipes to help you reduce fat consumption are provided at the end of this chapter

THE PROBLEM OF OVEREATING

Although there is still debate over whether obesity is a specific risk factor for a heart attack, the Framingham Heart Study and other long-term epidemiologic studies have found that overweight people, as a whole, have a higher incidence of heart disease. Since obesity contributes to high blood pressure and diabetes—both risk factors for heart disease—there is some scientific disagreement over whether obesity that occurs independently of either of these two health problems has an adverse effect on the heart. It is known, however, that obesity increases the heart's work load, since it entails an increase in total blood volume. In addition, excess weight puts undue stress on the joints, especially the knees, hips, and ankles, making it more difficult to maintain physical fitness.

A good deal is still unknown about why some people are obese and others, with similar background and food habits, are of normal weight. Recent studies indicate that some overweight people, especially habitual dieters, use food more efficiently and will therefore gain weight even when consuming fewer calories than their normal-weight counterparts. The theory is that their bodies have adjusted their metabolic thermostats, so to speak, at a lower level. For example, when crash dieting, the body adjusts to the lower food intake in much the same manner that it adjusts to threatened starvation. Everything, including metabolism, slows down to conserve energy. When deprived of food long enough, the dieter will lose weight, but the rate of weight loss drops. When he or she resumes a normal diet, the metabolism remains at a somewhat slower level and therefore the weight will go back up, even though calorie consumption may be within a range that normally would maintain ideal weight. This does not seem to happen if the dieting provides for a slow, steady weight loss—say two or three pounds a week—and is accompanied by an increase in physical activity.

THE QUESTION OF SALT

Ordinary table salt is made up of two minerals: sodium and chlorine (or sodium chloride in the combined form). We all need sodium chloride to maintain the balance of body fluids and to perform a number of essential body functions, including the conduction of nerve impulses, muscle contraction, and enzyme activity for digestion and food metabolism. But only very small amounts are needed; we can get by nicely on about five hundred to a thousand milligrams of sodium, or the amount in about one eighth to one fourth of a teaspoon of salt. The average American, however, consumes many times this amount of salt: 10 to 20 grams a day, or 2 to 4 teaspoons. (Five grams of salt equals about one teaspoon.) Ordinarily the kidneys eliminate the extra salt via the urine. Some people, however, consume more salt than their kidneys can excrete, causing an increase in body fluids. This increase in fluid volume causes the heart and the kidneys to work harder, and is thought to be one of the contributing factors in the development of high blood pressure.

The precise role excessive sodium consumption plays in high blood pressure is unknown. Epidemiologic studies of societies that consume very little salt have found that the people have virtually no hypertension. In contrast, societies that have a high salt intake—the Japanese and the Americans, for example—have a high incidence of hypertension. Animal studies have found that high blood pressure can be induced by a high-salt diet, particularly in strains that are genetically susceptible.

Our taste for salt seems to be an acquired one; we can get all the sodium we need from a balanced diet and our drinking water. But, from an early age, we tend to liberally season our food with salt, so even very young children soon acquire a taste for it, and often end up craving foods that are high in salt. In addition, salt is a hidden ingredient in many foods, particularly breakfast cereals, baked goods, canned vegetables and soups, processed meats, cheese, and many other common foods. Many people have the salt-shaker habit, liberally salting food before even tasting it. Whether or not sodium actually causes high blood pressure remains unknown. We do know, however, that restricting the salt intake of people with high blood pressure can lower the pressure. In fact, before the development of modern antihypertensive drugs, a major treatment for high blood pressure was strict limitation of sodium. Dr. Walter Kempner, a Duke physician known for his famous rice-and-fruit diet, was one of the first to treat a particularly lethal type of high blood pressure known as malignant hypertension with sodium restriction. Today, many people with mild hypertension can control their blood pressure through salt restriction, exercise, and, if needed, weight reduction. In others, reducing sodium intake seems to increase the effectiveness of antihypertensive drugs, meaning they can be taken at lower dosages, thereby reducing potential side effects. Reduced sodium intake is also important for patients with congestive heart failure or other disorders marked by fluid retention (edema).

THE ROLE OF FIBER

Dietary fiber, or roughage, is the undigestible portion of plant foods. It includes such things as the bran from cereal grains, pectin in apples and other fruits, and cellulose, which gives plants their structure. Until a decade ago, its importance in the human diet was largely ignored by nutritionists, because it does not contain any vitamins, minerals, or other nutrients that can be extracted by our digestive system.

Then came the studies of Denis P. Burkitt, a British physician who gained fame for his investigation of a type of cancer—Burkitt's lymphoma—that occurs mostly among young Africans. In the course of these studies, he noted that rural Africans were amazingly free of many of the diseases that are common in more industrialized societies—particularly colon cancers and other bowel disorders, and heart attacks. After studying the many differences in life-styles between the rural societies of many emerging nations and industrialized urban populations, Dr. Burkitt concluded that diet was one of the major factors. The rural societies tended to consume large amounts of fruits, vegetables, and unprocessed cereal grains—a diet that provided large amounts of dietary fiber—while the urban societies consumed a high-fat, high-meat diet with refined flour and grains from which the bran had been removed, and relatively little in the way of fruits and vegetables.

Since then, a number of studies have been undertaken to more precisely define the role of dietary fiber. Since fiber absorbs water as it moves through the digestive tract, it tends to produce a bulkier and softer stool, which moves more rapidly through the intestines. This reduced transit time is now thought to be important in protecting the colon against cancer from prolonged contact with some of the by-products of fat metabolism. It also reduces the tendency to constipation and is now considered to prevent the development of diverticulosis: small pockets that form along weakened segments of the colon wall.

The possible role of fiber in preventing heart disease is not as clear. Some studies have shown that a high-fiber diet may promote excretion of cholesterol in the stool, but whether this is a major factor in lowering blood cholesterol is not known. However, a high-fiber diet tends to be lower in total calories than one high in meat, fats, and refined carbohydrates. Therefore, fiber is a potentially important aid in losing excess weight. And since a high-fiber diet helps satisfy hunger by making you feel full, even though you have consumed fewer calories, it's also an aid in maintaining ideal weight.

THE DUPAC APPROACH TO A HEALTHFUL DIET

The first step in adopting a more healthful way of eating is to carefully analyze your present food habits, and then to determine what needs changing. As noted earlier, relatively few Americans are actually undernourished, even though their diet may not provide the right balance of nutrients. Deficiency diseases such as scurvy and rickets are very unusual in this country; we are much more likely to see problems related to excesses: obesity and high cholesterol are the two leading examples.

Very often, people who have had a heart attack feel almost betrayed when they learn that their diet may have been a contributing factor. Most of us eat what we like, and most of us think we have a basically healthful diet, even though we may admit to occasional overindulgence. Being told you should change the way you eat can, as Bob (the DUPAC patient described earlier in this chapter) put it, "seem like the final blow. . . . You have visions of giving up everything you like and living the rest of your life on a skimpy, tasteless diet."

It should be a pleasant surprise, then, to learn that it does not have to be this way. Following a DUPAC diet can be satisfying and tasty, as well as being good for you. It may mean modifying the way you shop and cook, but it does not mean forgoing everything you like (unless, of course, you like only a very few foods).

All DUPAC participants have the option of eating all their weekday meals in the DUPAC cafeteria, a new facility overlooking the Duke track and football field. There they have a wide selection of foods, attractively displayed and well prepared, that are low in calories, salt, and fat. (Other Duke programs, such as the Diet Rehabilitation Clinic, may be recommended for patients who are markedly overweight.)

Upon enrolling in DUPAC, patients have several sessions with a registered dietitian. If their spouses are available, they also may be included in these sessions. Patients are instructed to keep detailed food records of everything they eat and drink; when, where, and with whom they eat; and any activities, such as watching TV or working, that are associated with the eating. Many people are surprised to learn just how much they consume in the course of the day, and also about unexpected sources of calories. For example, John, a thirty-nine-year-old heart-attack patient, really thought he was sticking to his twelve-hundred-calorie-a-day diet. But he wasn't losing the expected two or more pounds a week. He was eating all the right things: small portions, lots of salads without dressing, no sweet desserts. But he totally overlooked the fact that during an average day he consumed six or more twelve-ounce bottles of regular soft drinks—an additional eight hundred or so calories a day. He switched to a diet drink and began losing the desired amount.

The circumstances of eating, particularly snacking and eating in restaurants, also is important. Many people do well when eating at home or in a controlled setting, such as the DUPAC cafeteria, but then lose control when eating in a restaurant, with business associates, or while traveling. Learning how to keep a Food Intake Record (see sample) and then planning for situations that are likely to tempt you to forget your dietary guidelines are important factors in altering faulty eating habits. An infrequent indiscretion is probably not going to matter too much in the long run, but people who frequently eat in restaurants or situations that are conducive to "breaking rules" should learn how to apply sound dietary principles to their life-styles.

In the DUPAC program, each participant has a dietary regimen designed to fit his or her individual eating habits, food preferences, and special medical problems, such as high blood pressure, overweight, or elevated cholesterol. In general, the diet is one that is low in calories and restricted in high-salt and high-cholesterol foods. Sample menus and recipes are made available, and one of the DUPAC dietitians is on hand in the DUPAC cafeteria to answer questions and offer advice. Since many of the DUPAC participants eat together, they also share their problems with each other and draw support from fellow patients. "It helps knowing you're not the only one in this situation," Bob told us. "I feel hungry most of the time, but when I eat with the others, I don't feel like I'm being deprived."

SIX IMPORTANT EATING TIPS

DUPAC dietitians have found that many of their patients, especially those who are overweight, have certain eating patterns that contribute to their weight problems. For example, they tend to eat quickly. Many find it impossible to leave anything on their plates; still others are frequent snackers. To help correct these faulty habits, DUPAC tables are set with reminder cards designed to reinforce several good eating practices. These include:

1. Plan a pause during your meal. Uninterrupted eating leads to overeating. That's why it's an excellent practice to plan a two- or three-minute pause at about the midpoint in your meal. This gives your body a chance to "catch up," so you'll begin to feel full. Some dieters time their pause with an egg timer or electric food timer. It doesn't matter. The important thing is to take a two- or three-minute break. You'll eat less and feel fuller.

2. Always put your fork down between bites. This will help you establish a slower pace of eating. And that means you'll enjoy your meal more: feel more satisfied when you are finished. It's a small technique, but it will help you be more conscious of what and how much you are eating. Remember: when your fork is on your plate, you aren't stuffing yourself with calories.

3. Don't prepare the next bite while you're still chewing one. Take your time. Eating wasn't meant to be a race. So slow down. You'll feel fuller even though you've eaten less.

4. Remove serving dishes from the table. After everyone has helped himself, it's a good idea to remove the serving dishes. That way, you put temptation behind you. And when your goal is to lose weight, every temptation avoided is a victory won. What you don't see, you don't want. What you don't want, you don't eat. What you don't eat, you don't have to lose.

5. Establish one place in the house that is the only place where you eat. Many a diet goes astray because we've become accustomed to eating all over the house. If you're serious about dieting, this "snacking pattern" should be changed. Associate eating with only one place and eat only there. Chances are you'll cut down your caloric intake considerably by just restricting your opportunities.

6. Mark off a small portion of something you especially like at the beginning of the meal—then leave it. We all tend to go overboard on certain foods. The best way to handle this situation is by defusing the trap before it grabs us. And the easiest way is simply to set aside a small portion of your favorite food and then leave that portion on the plate. You'll feel better for it.

PUTTING THE PRINCIPLES INTO PRACTICE

On the following pages, you will find the complete eating plan that is recommended for most DUPAC heart patients who are moderately overweight. The accompanying recipes give the total calories per serving and other important nutritional information. A sample Food Intake Record that you can use to keep track of what you eat and drink and the circumstances involved is also included. Most DUPAC patients find this record particularly useful in identifying forgotten sources of calories, such as large numbers of soft drinks consumed throughout the day, or circumstances in which they are apt to stray from the recommended diet, for example snacking while watching TV or when meeting business associates. The Nutritional History is helpful in identifying problems that should be corrected, as well as providing a record of dietary recommendations from your own doctor or dietitian.

SUMMING UP

What we eat is obviously an important factor in maintaining total health. The traditional American diet—high in meat, fat, salt, and sugar, and relatively low in fruits and vegetables—may well influence the development of several cardiovascular risk factors, particularly high cholesterol, high blood pressure, and obesity. Modifying your eating habits to bring them in line with the prudent approach recommended for DUPAC patients and endorsed by the American Heart Association is a commonsense approach to achieving total health.

DUKE UNIVERSITY MEDICAL CENTER
NUTRITIONAL HISTORY

Age:_____   Sex:_____   Marital Status:_____
Ht.:_____   Wt.:_____   Ideal Weight:_____
Diagnosis:_____
Medications:_____
Present Activity Level:_____
Occupation:_____
Hours of Work:_____
Laboratory Values:
    Cholesterol_____ Triglycerides_____ HDL_____ LDL_____
    Glucose_____ Other_____
BMR (Basal metabolic rate):_____ Activity Factor_____
Have you been following a special diet at home?_____
What kinds of diets have you followed in the past?_____
Who prepares your meals?_____
Frequency of restaurant dining?_____
Food allergies?_____
Appetite change?_____
Weight History: 18 years old   _____
                    1 year ago   _____
                    Highest adult weight _____
                    Lowest adult weight _____
                    Patient goal   _____
                    Present weight   _____
                                    _____
                                    _____
                                    _____
                                    _____
                                    _____

Typical Daily Food Intake
List all foods and beverages, and the amounts and times eaten.

Estimated Daily Intake:
    Calories_____ Protein_____ Carbohydrate_____ Fat_____
    Sodium_____ Saturated_____ Unsaturated_____

Recommendations:
    Calories_____ Protein_____ Carbohydrate_____ Fat_____
    Sodium_____ Saturated_____ Unsaturated_____

1. _____
2. _____
3. _____
4. _____
5. _____

Date   *Comments:*

DAILY FOOD INTAKE RECORD

Date: _____   Name: _____

Time Start/End	Place	Alone or with whom?	Associated activity	Food/ Amount	Calories
6–11 A.M.					
11 A.M.– 4 P.M.					
4–9 P.M.					
9 P.M.–6 A.M.					

CHOLESTEROL CONTENT OF FOODS

Food	Household Measure	Cholesterol in Mgs.
Beef, composite of retail cuts, cooked	3 oz.	80
Brains, raw	3 oz.	1690
Butter, regular	1 T.	35
Buttermilk, nonfat	1c.	5
Cake, homemade chocolate with frosting	1/16 of 9″ diam.	32
angel food	1/12 of 10″ diam.	0
sponge	1/12 of 10″ diam.	162
Caviar, sturgeon	1 T.	48
Cheese, Cheddar	1 oz.	28
cottage, 1% fat	1/4 c.	6
mozzarella, part skim	1 oz.	18
processed American cheese food	1 oz.	20
Chicken, composite of flesh and skin	3 oz.	74
Clams, canned, drained	3 oz.	54
Crab, canned, drained	3 oz.	86
Cream, heavy whipping	1 T.	20
half-and-half	1 T.	6
sour	1 T.	8
Eggs, whole	1 large	252
white only	1	0
Fish, fresh	3 oz.	45
salmon, canned	3 oz.	30
sardines, canned, in oil	3 oz.	102
tuna, canned, in oil	3 oz.	47
Frankfurter, cooked	1 frank	34
Gizzard, composite, cooked	3 oz.	180
Heart, composite, cooked	3 oz.	211
Ice cream, 10% fat	1 c.	53
Ice milk	1 c.	26
Kidneys, composite, cooked	3 oz.	683
Lamb, composite, cooked	3 oz.	83
Lard	1 T.	12
Liver, composite of large animals	3 oz.	372
poultry	3 oz.	572
Lobster, cooked	3 oz.	72
Margarine, all vegetable fat	1 T.	0
Mayonnaise	1 T.	10
Milk, whole	1 c.	34
2% fat	1 c.	22
skim	1 c.	5
Noodles, egg, cooked	1 c.	50
Oysters, canned solids and liquid	3 oz.	38
Pies, baked custard	1/8 of 9″ diam.	120
fruit	1/8 of 9″ diam.	0

Food	Household Measure	Cholesterol in Mgs.
Pork, composite of lean retail cuts	3 oz.	76
Scallops, steamed	3 oz.	45
Shrimp, canned, drained	3 oz.	128
Sweetbreads, cooked	3 oz.	396
Turkey, cooked flesh and skin	3 oz.	79
Veal, composite, cooked	3 oz.	86
Yogurt, nonfat plain or vanilla	8 oz.	17

DUPAC'S WEIGHT-REDUCTION DIET

The following meal plans provide for a balanced 1,000-calorie-per-day eating plan. The menus are those served in the DUPAC cafeteria and cover three 5-day cycles. Most of the dishes served are common favorites that can be found in most general cookbooks or *The American Heart Association Cookbook*. Calories can be cut out of most recipes by reducing the amount of fat and by substituting low-calorie ingredients for high-calorie counterparts, such as skim milk instead of whole milk. Weekend meals can be repeats of a meal during the week, or can be constructed from the special DUPAC recipes included here.

DUPAC 1,000-Calorie Meal Plan

Suggested menus:

Breakfast

	Calories
1 box cereal (or 1/2 c. hot cereal)	75
1/2 c. skim milk	50
1 serving fruit	40
1 T. raisins	20
	185
3/4 c. cottage cheese	150
1 serving fruit	40
	190
2 egg whites	30
1/2 t. corn oil (used in prep.)	20
1/4 c. cottage cheese	50
1 serving fruit	40
	140

(To be served Monday, Wednesday, and Friday)

Breakfast

	Calories
1 c. muesli	170
1/2 c. skim milk	50
	220
2/3 c. plain yogurt	100
1 serving fruit	40
4 oz. orange juice	40
	180
1/2 pita bread	70
(white or wheat)	
Egg Beaters (60	100
gm.)	170

(To be served Tuesday,
Thursday, and
Saturday)

1 waffle	90
1 serving fruit	40
1/2 c. skim milk	50
	180

(To be served Sunday)

Standard substitutions:
–Dry cereals: See Calorie Content List
–Raw, unprocessed bran: 10 calories per tablespoon
–Hot cereals: 75 calories per 1/2 cup
    Oatmeal   Cream of Wheat
    Pettijohns   Grits
–Fruits: fresh (a variety), canned unsweetened (peaches, pineapple), and
    dried (raisins). Average calorie value is 40 per 1/2 cup or 1/2 fruit.
    Raisins have 20 calories per tablespoon.
–High-protein foods:
    Egg whites: 25 calories each (15 for egg, 10 for 1/4 teaspoon corn oil)
    Plain yogurt: 50 calories per 1/3 cup

Cottage cheese: 50 calories per 1/4 cup
Vanilla or lemon yogurt: 50 calories per 1/4 cup
–Bran muffins, blueberry muffins: 110 calories each

CALORIE CONTENT
FOR DRY CEREALS

All-Bran	90	Raisin Bran	120
All-Bran Flakes	90	Rice Krispies	70
Cheerios	80	Shredded Wheat	90
Cornflakes	80	Special K	70
Puffed rice	40	Total	110
Puffed wheat	35		

DUPAC 1,000-Calorie Meal Plan

	MONDAY		TUESDAY	
Lunch	*Item*	*Calories*	*Item*	*Calories*
	Garden Vegetable Salad:		Tuna and Cottage Cheese in Tomato:	
	3 tomato slices	30	3 oz. light tuna	105
	1/2 c. cottage cheese w/shredded carrots, onion, green pepper	100	1/4 c. cottage cheese	50
			tomato	20
	3 cucumber slices		Lettuce bed	0
	3 celery sticks			175
	2 carrot sticks	15		
		145	1 c. vegetable soup	40
			1/2 c. unsweetened pineapple chunks*	40
	1 T. low-calorie French dressing	25	2 Melba Toast	30
	1 c. chili	100		285
	1/2 c. unsweetened peach halves	40	* Fresh fruit may be substituted	
		310		
Dinner	*Item*	*Calories*	*Item*	*Calories*
	Tuna Casserole	195	5 oz. sirloin steak	300
	w/2 oz. mushroom sauce	75	1/3 c. corn	70
	1/2 c. peas & carrots	45	1/2 c. green beans	25
	1/2 c. tomatoes	20	2 tomato slices on lettuce leaf	20
	Small tossed salad	10	1 dinner roll	80
	1/2–1 oz. light dressing	15		495
	Fresh fruit	40		
	1 dinner roll	80	Substitute:	
		480	6 oz. chicken	
	Substitute: 6 oz. chicken (must omit 30 cal.)			

Week I

WEDNESDAY		THURSDAY		FRIDAY	
Item	*Calories*	*Item*	*Calories*	*Item*	*Calories*
Apple Salad:		Hot Open-		Salad Bar	
1/2 c. vanilla yogurt	100	Faced Roast		(select items to	
1/2 c. diced apple	40	Beef Sandwich:		add up to	
1 T. raisins	20	2 oz. lean roast		180 cal.)	180
1 T. celery	5	beef	120	2 T. low-calorie	
1/4 t. cinnamon	0	1 sl. white or		dressing	40
	165	wheat bread	70	1 c. vegetable soup	40
		1 oz. gravy	10		260
1 c. chili	100		200		
1/2 c. unsweetened				(Calories may vary	
pears	40	1 c. vegetable soup	40	according to the	
	305	1/2 c. fresh fruit		dressing you	
		cup	40	choose.)	
			280		
				Substitute:	
				1 c. chili	100

Item	*Calories*	*Item*	*Calories*	*Item*	*Calories*
6 oz. Lemon Baked		4 oz. turkey	200	6 oz. chicken with	
Chicken	300	1 oz. turkey gravy	10	Rosemary	300
1/4 acorn squash	40	1/2 c. asparagus	25	1/2 c. spinach	25
1/2 c. Italian-style		1 potato	90	1/2 c. mushrooms	25
mixed vegetables		1/2 c. carrot-raisin-		1/2 c. mashed potato	90
(green beans,		pineapple salad	75	2 oz. gravy	20
onions, zucchini,		2 c. tossed salad	20	1/2 c. Jell-O	45
broccoli, tomatoes)	25	1 oz. Lemon Yogurt			505
		topping or	25		
Fresh fruit	40	2 T. low-calorie		Substitute:	
1 dinner roll	80	dressing	40	5 oz. roast beef	
	485		445		
			or 460		
Substitute:					
6 oz. turkey					

DUPAC 1,000-Calorie Meal Plan

	MONDAY		TUESDAY	
Lunch	*Item*	*Calories*	*Item*	*Calories*
	1 c. chili	100	1 c. vegetable soup	40
	1/2 c. chicken salad:		Turkey cold	
	1 oz. chicken	50	plate:	
	2 T. egg white	10	2 oz. sliced	
	2 T. onion	10	turkey	100
	2 T. celery	10	1 oz. beef	60
	1/2 oz. light		2 tomato slices	20
	dressing	_25_	5 cucumber slices	5
		105	1/2 –1 oz. light	
			dressing	_15_
	6 white asparagus			200
	spears	25		
	2 tomato slices	_20_	2 Melba Toast	30
		150	1 fresh fruit	_40_
				310
	1/2 c. unsweetened			
	apricots	_40_		
		290		
Dinner	*Item*	*Calories*	*Item*	*Calories*
	5 oz. turbot	300	5 oz. sirloin	
	1/2 c. carrots	25	steak	300
	1/2 baked potato	45	1/2 potato	45
	1/2 c. slaw	15	1/2 c. asparagus	25
	1/2 oz. light		fresh fruit	40
	dressing	25	1 dinner roll	_80_
	1/2 c. pears	_40_		490
		450		
			Substitute:	
	Substitute:		6 oz. chicken	
	6 oz. chicken			

Week II

WEDNESDAY		THURSDAY		FRIDAY	
Item	*Calories*	*Item*	*Calories*	*Item*	*Calories*
1 c. chili	100	Stuffed baked		Salad bar	
		potato	90	(select items to	
Vegetable pita:		w/stir-		add up to	
1/4 c. cottage		fried vegetables		180 cal.)	180
cheese	50	(1/2 c.)	50		
4 cucumber slices	---	and Cheese		2 T. low-calorie	
4 carrot slices	---	(1 oz.)	100	dressing	40
4 slices tomato	25		240		
Shredded lettuce	---			1 c. vegetable soup	40
2 T. dill dressing	40	1/2 c. unsweetened		(Calories may vary	
1/2 pita bread	80	peach halves	40	according to the	
	195		280	dressing you	
	295			choose.)	
					260
				Substitute:	
				1 c. chili	100

Item	*Calories*	*Item*	*Calories*	*Item*	*Calories*
1 c. vegetable soup	40	6 oz. chicken	300	4 oz. turkey	200
6 oz. baked		w/ 2 T. Parmesan		1 oz. turkey gravy	10
flounder	210	Herb Mixture	35	1/2 c. broccoli	
w/1 pat		1/2 c. vegetable		soufflé	75
margarine	45	medley: (squash,		1/2 c. yellow	
1/2 stuffed potato	95	green beans, carrots,		squash	25
1 c. broccoli	50	onions)	25	Small salad w/	
1/2 c. Jell-O	45	1/2 c. mashed		2 tomato slices	20
	485	potatoes	90	1/2–1 oz. light	
		1/4 c. peaches	20	dressing	15
Substitute:		1 oz. vanilla yogurt		Fresh fruit	40
6 oz. chicken		for peaches	25	1 dinner roll	80
(must omit 90 cal.)			495	1 pat margarine	45
					510
		Substitute:			
		5 oz. turbot		Substitute:	
				6 oz. chicken	
				(must omit 100 cal.)	

DUPAC 1,000-Calorie Meal Plan

	MONDAY		TUESDAY	
	Item	*Calories*	*Item*	*Calories*
Lunch	1 c. chili	100	1/2 c. chicken salad:	
			1 oz. chicken	50
	1/2 c. carrot-pineapple-		2 T. egg white	10
	raisin salad	75	2 T. onion	10
	1 oz. lemon yogurt	25	2 T. celery	10
	1/4 c. cottage cheese	50	1/2 oz. light	
	1 tomato slice	10	dressing	25
	1 fresh fruit	40		105
		300	6 asparagus spears	20
			2 tomato slices	20
				145
			1 whole wheat roll	80
			1 pat margarine	45
				270
	Item	*Calories*	*Item*	*Calories*
Dinner	Stuffed pepper	300	4 oz. roast pork	240
	1/2 c. yellow squash	25	1/2 c. cabbage	25
	1/2 c. French-style		1/2 c. green peas	70
	green beans	25	Small salad	10
	Small salad	10	1/2–1 oz. light	
	w/2 tomato wedges	20	dressing	15
	1/2–1 oz. light		1/4 c. pineapple	20
	dressing	15	1 oz. lemon yogurt	
		395	topping	25
				405
	Substitute:			
	6 oz. chicken		Substitute:	
			6 oz. chicken	
			(must omit 60 cal.)	

Week III

	WEDNESDAY	THURSDAY		FRIDAY	

Item	Calories	Item	Calories	Item	Calories
1 c. vegetable soup	40	1 c. chili	100	Salad bar:	
Cold plate:		Garden vegetable		(select items to	
1 oz. turkey	50	salad:		add up to	
1 oz. roast beef	60	3 tomato slices	30	180 cal.)	180
2 tomato slices	20	1/2 c. cottage		2 T. low-calorie	
Small salad	10	cheese	100	dressing	40
1/2–1 oz. light		w/shredded carrots,		1 c. vegetable	
dressing	15	onions, green		soup	40
2 Melba Toast	30	pepper,			260
1 fresh fruit	40	3 carrots,		(Calories may vary	
	265	3 celery sticks	15	according to the	
				dressing you	
		1/2 c. unsweetened		choose.)	
		fruit cocktail	40		
			285	Substitute:	
				1 c. chili	100

Item	Calories	Item	Calories	Item	Calories
4 oz. turkey	200	6 oz. Italian		Beef loaf	
2 oz. turkey gravy	10	Flounder	255	casserole	220
1/2 stuffed potato	95	1/2 c. zucchini	25	1/4 pineapple acorn	
1/2 c. spinach	25	1/2 c. corn	70	squash	75
1/2 c. mushrooms	25	Small salad	10	1/2 c. green beans	25
Fresh fruit	40	1/2–1 oz. light		1/2 c. slaw	15
	395	dressing	15	1 oz. light	
			375	dressing	25
Substitute:				1/2 baked apple	40
6 oz. chicken		Substitute:			400
(must omit 100 cal.)		6 oz. chicken			
		(must omit 45 cal.)		Substitute:	
				6 oz. chicken	
				(must omit 80 cal.)	

DUPAC RECIPES

Breakfast

EGG-WHITE CREPE

3 egg whites	45 cal.
1/2 T. corn-oil margarine	50 cal.

Beat egg whites until frothy. Fry in margarine. Turn once.
Use any of the following for filling:
1. Sprinkle with cinnamon and Sweet 'n Low. Roll as you would any crepe.
2. Spread a small amount of diet jelly or marmalade on crepe. Roll as you would any crepe.
(1 serving)   95 cal. per serving

COTTAGE APPLESAUCE

1 c. skim-milk cottage cheese
2 c. unsweetened applesauce
Dash of cinnamon or nutmeg

Mix cottage cheese and applesauce. Chill.
Garnish with orange slice.
(4 servings)   80 cal. per serving

EGG WHITES

3 egg whites (separate)		45 cal.
1/2 T. corn-oil margarine		<u>50 cal.</u>
	Total	95 cal.

Melt margarine in frying pan. Cook each egg white separately (looks like a small pancake). Turn egg to cook on other side.
You may then take 1/4 c. cottage cheese and layer egg whites with cottage cheese. Total: 145 cal.

Soups

PREPARATION OF STOCK

1. *Beef Stock*

   Place beef and beef bones in large pot. Cover with water and bring to a boil. Reduce heat and simmer 1 hour. Set aside until cool. Remove meat and bones.

   Strain into another pot and place in refrigerator overnight. Next day remove *all* of the solidified fat from top of stock.

2. *Chicken Stock*

   Boil chicken for at least 1 hour. Set aside to cool. Remove chicken from broth. Strain into another pot and place in refrigerator overnight. Next day, remove *all* of the solidified fat from top of stock.

3. Using either the chicken or beef stock, proceed as follows. Add

   2 c. diced celery
   2 c. diced onions
   2 c. diced carrots
   4 c. chopped cabbage
   1 sm. can tomato paste
   4 c. diced tomatoes

   Simmer at low heat for 30 minutes. Season with favorite spices. Divide into portions and freeze.

   1½ oz. chicken added to 12 oz. soup totals approx. 150 cal.

VEGETABLE SOUP VARIATIONS

CLAM CHOWDER

8 oz. soup	55 cal.
½ c. cooked clams	78 cal.
Total	133 cal.

Season with thyme. Serve hot!

CRAB GUMBO

8 oz. soup		55 cal.
1/4 c. okra		17 cal.
3 oz. crabmeat		85 cal.
	Total	157 cal.

Serve hot!

Salad & Salad Dressings

APPLE SALAD

3 medium-sized firm apples (cored and diced fine)
3 c. finely shredded cabbage
1 T. prepared horseradish
6 T. low-calorie French dressing

Combine apples and cabbage. Mix horseradish and diet dressing and then pour over apples and cabbage.

(6 servings)   60 cal. per serving.

PEPPY SPICY COLESLAW

1 8-ounce can fruit cocktail (rinse in water to remove syrup)	100 cal.
2 c. shredded red cabbage	32 cal.
2 c. shredded white cabbage	32 cal.

Mix together cabbages and fruit
  cocktail

1/2 c. plain yogurt	65 cal.
2 t. mustard	–
1/2 t. ginger	–
Total	229 cal.

Mix dressing
  Add dressing to salad.
  (8 servings)   Approx. 30 cal. per serving.

CUCUMBER SALAD

1 large cucumber		29 cal.
1/4 med. onion		10 cal.
Vinegar Dressing		0 cal.
	Total	39 cal.

GREEN BEAN SALAD

1/2 c. cooked string beans		15 cal.
1/4 med. onion		10 cal.
Vinegar Dressing		0 cal.
	Total	25 cal.

DIET COLESLAW

Finely shredded cabbage
Finely shredded carrot
Finely shredded green pepper
Vinegar Dressing (celery seed
  may be added if desired)

  Total per 1/2 cup: 15 cal.

SPINACH SALAD

1/2 c. raw spinach		20 cal.
1 chopped egg white		15 cal.
1 oz. diet French dressing		30 cal.
	Total	65 cal.

BEET SALAD

1/2 c. cooked beets		25 cal.
1/4 med. onion		10 cal.
Vinegar dressing		0 cal.
	Total	35 cal.

*BEET AND COTTAGE CHEESE SALAD

1 env. unflav. gelatin		28 cal.
2 pks. Sweet 'n Low		0 cal.
1 1/2 c. water		
1/4 c. lemon juice		24 cal.
1 c. chopped cooked beets		50 cal.
1 c. cottage cheese		200 cal.
	Total	302 cal.

(6 servings)   50 cal. per serving

*PERFECTION SALAD

1 env. unflav. gelatin		28 cal.
1 pk. Sweet 'n Low		0 cal.
1 1/4 c. water (divided)		
1 T. lemon juice		8 cal.
1/2 c. shredded cabbage		15 cal.
1 c. chopped celery		20 cal.
1/2 red pepper, chopped		8 cal.
1/2 green pepper, chopped		8 cal.
	Total	87 cal.

(4 servings)   22 cal. per serving

* Mixing method for gelatin salads
Mix gelatin and Sweet 'n Low in a saucepan. Add 1/2 c. water and stir constantly until dissolved. Remove from heat and stir in remaining water and juice. Chill to consistency of unbeaten egg white. Fold in other ingredients. Chill until set.

Vinegar Dressing—0 cal.

Put 1¹/2 c. vinegar into a pint jar. Add ¹/2 c. water and 1¹/2 pks. of Sweet 'n Low. Shake. This may be kept in refrigerator and used as needed.

Yogurt Dill Dressing

¹/2 c. low-fat yogurt
¹/2 c. low-calorie mayonnaise
¹/2 T. dill weed
2 T. skim milk

Combine and chill. Makes just over 1 cup. 20 calories per 1-tablespoon serving

Hot Green Bean Salad

¹/4 c. diet Italian dressing
2 pks. (9 oz. each) frozen cut green
  beans
¹/2 c. diced celery
1 large onion (cut into rings and
  separated)
2 t. dried dill weed

Cook green beans. Drain. In same pan with beans add Italian dressing, celery, onion, and dill. Cook for 3 minutes, stirring occasionally. Be sure it does not dry out while cooking. If so, add 1 tablespoon water.

Carbohydrate 12 gm.　Protein 2 gm.　Fat negligible.

(6 servings)　37 cal. per serving.

Green Salad Mold

1 env. unflav. gelatin	28 cal.
1 pk. Sweet 'n Low	0 cal.
1/8 t. pepper	0 cal.
13/4 c. water—divided	0 cal.
1/4 c. vinegar	9 cal.
1 T. lemon juice	8 cal.
6 sm. green onions	40 cal.
1 c. raw shredded spinach	40 cal.
1 c. chopped celery	20 cal.
1/4 c. shredded carrot	10 cal.
Total	155 cal.

(6 servings)   26 cal. per serving

Waldorf Salad

1 env. unflav. gelatin	28 cal.
2 pks. Sweet 'n Low	0 cal.
11/2 c. water	0 cal.
1/4 c. lemon juice	24 cal.
3 apples, diced	225 cal.
1/2 c. chopped celery	10 cal.
Total	287 cal.

(6 servings)   48 cal. per serving

Fruit Salad Dressing

4 T. lemon juice
1/2 c. orange juice
1/4 t. paprika
dash nutmeg
dietary salt substitute to taste

Combine all ingredients and blend well. Chill. Shake before using.
Makes 3/4 c. (72 cal.)   1 T. supplies 6 calories.

Main Dishes

Egg White	Beef
Fish	Veal
Chicken	Lamb

OMELET

3 egg whites	45 cal.
1/2 onion	20 cal.
1/2 green pepper	5 cal.
1/2 c. mushrooms	20 cal.
1/4 c. cottage cheese	50 cal.
1/2 T. corn-oil margarine	50 cal.
1/2 c. Basic Tomato Sauce	50 cal.
Total	240 cal.

Beat egg whites until light and frothy. Fry egg whites in corn oil until firm, turning once. Remove eggs to warm plate. In same pan, sauté onion, green pepper, and mushrooms. Add 1/4 cup tomato sauce. Cook until vegetables are tender. Place the mixture on one half of omelet, along with the cottage cheese. Fold omelet. Heat remaining tomato sauce and pour it over omelet.

DUPAC CHILI

8 oz. beef, lean
1/2 c. onion, diced
1/2 c. green pepper, diced
4 c. fresh mushrooms, sliced
1 T. chili powder
1 T. dry parsley
1 t. oregano
1/4 t. garlic powder
1/4 t. black pepper
4 12-oz. cans unsalted tomato juice

Brown beef, then add all other ingredients. Simmer for 2 to 2½ hours. Serves 6–8, 100 calories per 8-ounce serving.

Scallops in White Wine

1¹/4 lbs. scallops
1 c. dry white wine
4 small white onions, chopped
1 clove garlic, minced
black pepper
chopped parsley

Place scallops in baking dish. Cover with onions, wine, and garlic. Sprinkle with pepper. Bake in preheated oven at 350° for 10 minutes, until scallops are done. Sprinkle chopped parsley over them. Garnish with lemon slices and paprika.

6 oz. scallops per serving (240 calories)

Each portion must be weighed at serving time. Scallops shrink during cooking.

Fat-free Fillets of Fish with Scalloped Potatoes and Onions

(You can use any lean white fish for this very simple but satisfying dish.)

1 large onion, very thinly sliced
1 cup each fish or chicken stock and no-fat skim milk (we used skim milk powder plus water); more if needed
4 medium-size "boiling" potatoes, very thinly sliced
Pepper and mixed herbs to taste (we used "Italian Seasoning")
About 1¹/4 lb. skinless and boneless lean fish fillets, such as cod, hake, haddock, sole, perch, whitefish, or even trout
2 T. fresh minced parsley

Simmer the sliced onion in a medium-sized saucepan with the stock and milk while you are peeling and slicing the potatoes; add the potatoes, pepper, and herbs to taste. Simmer, adding a little more liquid if needed to cover ingredients, for 7 to 8 minutes, or until potato slices are just tender. Meanwhile, trim the fish filets into serving-size pieces, and slice them horizontally, if necessary, to make them no more than 1/2 inch thick; season them lightly with salt, pepper, and herbs.

When potatoes and onions are tender, spread half of them in the bottom of a shallow flameproof baking and serving dish, arrange the fish over them, and cover with the remaining potatoes and onions. Pour on the cooking liquid, adding a little more of the stock or milk so that the ingredients are just barely covered.

About half an hour before you are ready to serve, preheat oven to 375° F. Cut a piece of waxed paper to fit top of dish, to keep the top from browning, and lay over the ingredients. Bring contents just to the simmer on top of the stove; then set in middle level of preheated oven. Bake for 15 minutes, basting twice with liquid in dish. Remove waxed paper, sprinkle on the parsley, and serve.

(4 servings)   320 calories per serving.

SHRIMP CREOLE

1/2 T. margarine or corn oil	50 cal.
2 med. green peppers	30 cal.
1 onion	40 cal.
1/2 c. chopped celery	10 cal.
1 can diet tomatoes	100 cal.
1 pk. Sweet 'n Low	0 cal.
1 t. chili powder	0 cal.
1 clove garlic or garlic powder	0 cal.
dash Tabasco	0 cal.
1 bay leaf	0 cal.
salt substitute to taste	
12 oz. shrimp	400 cal.
Total	630 cal.

In large skillet, sauté green peppers, onion, and celery until tender. Add tomatoes, Sweet 'n Low, chili powder, garlic, Tabasco, bay leaf, and salt substitute. Simmer for about 15 minutes. Add shrimp and continue simmering until shrimp are tender. Do not overcook. Serve over rice.

(4 servings)   160 calories per serving

1/2 cup rice = 100 calories, or 245 cal. per serving

1/2 c. diet coleslaw   15 cal.
baked apple   75 cal.
                 Total   335 cal. per serving

SAUCY HADDOCK BAKE

1 1/2 lb. haddock fillets	*2 t. grated onion*
2 T. corn-oil margarine (to grease	*1/8 t. pepper*
pan and dot over fish)	*1 bay leaf*
1 T. lemon juice	*chopped parsley*

Arrange fish fillets in greased shallow baking dish. Combine remaining ingredients and pour over fish and dot with remaining margarine. Bake at 400° F for 25 minutes or until fish flakes. Sprinkle with parsley and serve immediately.

Season with dietary salt substitute to taste.

(4 servings)   180 cal. per serving.

DIET "PIZZA"

1 1/2 c. cooked rice	300 cal.
1 egg white mixed with 1 T. water	15 cal.
1/2 lb. lean ground round steak	390 cal.
(cooks down to 6 oz.)	
1/2 c. finely diced green pepper	8 cal.
1/2 med. onion, finely diced	20 cal.
1 4-oz. can mushroom stems and	25 cal.
pieces	
1/2 c. cottage cheese	100 cal.
1/2 c. Basic Tomato Sauce	50 cal.
garlic powder to taste	
oregano to taste	
Total	908 cal.

Mix rice with egg-white mixture and press into 9" pie pan. Bake rice crust for 12 minutes at 450°. Remove from oven.

Brown ground steak in skillet. Drain all fat and spread the beef evenly in the rice crust. Sauté the pepper, onion, and mushrooms, using the pan the meat was cooked in. Add a little water if vegetables become too dry. Arrange vegetables over meat.

Spread 1/2 c. cottage cheese over vegetables and meat, and cover all with tomato sauce.

Sprinkle with garlic powder to taste. Add oregano to taste.

Bake 20 minutes at 350°.

(6 servings)   150 cal. per serving.

TASTY BEEF PATTIES

1 lb. lean ground beef (16 oz. will cook down to about 13 oz.)	845 cal.
1 4-oz. can mushroom stems and pieces (drained)	25 cal.
1 T. prepared mustard	
2 T. instant minced onions	negligible
1/2 t. garlic powder	
1/4 t. black pepper	
Total	870 cal.

Mix all ingredients. Shape into 6 patties.
145 cal. per pattie.

LAMB STEW

1 lb. lean lamb shoulder
1 T. margarine
1 c. sliced onion
1/4 t. coarse fresh black pepper
3/4 t. ground allspice
1/4 t. ground ginger
1 c. Basic Tomato Sauce
3 c. cooked carrots
1 1/2 c. water (about)

Cut lamb in 2″ cubes. Be sure to trim off all fat. Melt margarine in nonstick skillet. Add meat, and brown on all sides. Add onion, and brown lightly. Drain all fat that has accumulated in pan. Stir in pepper, allspice, ginger, and 1/2 a cup of the water. Cover, and simmer about 2 hours, adding more water if necessary. Remove any fat that appears with a bulb-type baster. Add tomato sauce and cooked carrots and cook about 15 minutes longer. Canned sliced carrots may be used, but be sure to rinse them well to remove salt. Season to taste with salt substitute.

(6 servings.)   Approx. 194 cal. per serving.*

Carbohydrate 10.7 gm. Protein 23.1 gm. Total fat 6.4 gm. (sat. fat 3.4) Cholesterol 75.7 mg.

* May be thickened with 1 T. cornstarch. Add 6 cal. per serving if cornstarch is used, for a total of 200 cal. per serving.

CoQ au Vin (Chicken in Burgundy)

3 whole boned chicken breasts
1 T. corn-oil margarine
1 c. beef stock (salt free)
1/2 c. burgundy
1 t. thyme
1 t. marjoram

2 T. chopped parsley
12 small white boiling onions,
*   peeled*
4 celery stalks, whole
1 T. cornstarch

Cut chicken breasts in half. Brown the chicken breasts on grill in margarine. Heat the beef stock and add it to the pan. Add wine, thyme, marjoram, parsley, and onions. Cover with celery stalks. Cook slowly for 1 hour over low heat. Discard celery stalks and remove chicken and onions to a serving dish. Measure pan juices and add more water if necessary to make 1 cup. Return to pan and add 1 tablespoon cornstarch (which has been mixed with water). Cook until thick. Add salt substitute to taste.

(6 servings)   190 cal. per serving.

CHICKEN BREAST CREOLE

1 large onion	*garlic powder*
2 green peppers	*black pepper*
2 T. margarine	*oregano*
2 lbs. chicken breast	*thyme*
without skin and bone	*1 1/2 c. dry white wine*
1 c. mushrooms	*3 c. canned tomatoes*
onion powder	

Chop onion and green pepper. Melt margarine in nonstick skillet. Add chicken, and brown on both sides. Remove to a platter.

Add onions, mushrooms, and green peppers to the pan and sauté until soft and golden brown. Return chicken to pan. Add onion powder, garlic powder, pepper, oregano, and thyme according to your own taste. Add the wine and the tomatoes with tomato liquid. Cover and simmer 1 hour. Season to taste with salt substitute. Pan juices may be thickened with 1 tablespoon cornstarch.

(6 servings)   Approx. 244 cal. per serving.
Protein 29 gm. Carbohydrate 11 gm. Total fat 6 gm. (sat. fat 1.6 gm.)
Cholesterol 89.3 mg.

MOROCCAN CHICKEN

2 lb. fryer/broiler chicken quartered
and skinned
1 T. grated lemon peel
1/2 c. water
1/4 c. lemon juice
1 t. thyme
1 t. garlic powder
1/2 t. black pepper
1 lemon
1/4 c. chopped parsley

Combine the grated lemon peel, water, lemon juice, thyme, garlic powder, and pepper. Pour over chicken, coating it well. Refrigerate for 3–4 hours, turning the chicken in the marinade several times.

Arrange the chicken in a single layer in a shallow baking dish.

Save the liquid marinade. Bake the chicken uncovered at 425° for 25 minutes. Pour off any fat that has accumulated in the pan. Lower oven temperature to 350°. Brush chicken with the reserved marinade and bake 25–35 minutes, until the chicken is tender and brown. Cut the lemon into thin slices and serve the chicken with the lemon slices as garnish. Sprinkle parsley over completed dish.

(4 servings.)   222 cal. per serving.
Carbohydrate 1.5 gm. Protein 33 gm. Total fat 9 gm.

Season with dietary salt substitute to taste.

Vegetables

CARAWAY CARROTS

1 lb. cooked carrots
2 t. corn-oil margarine
2 T. lemon juice
1/2 t. grated lemon rind
1 t. caraway seed
pepper to taste
dietary salt substitute to taste

To hot cooked, drained carrots add corn-oil margarine, lemon juice and rind, and caraway seed. Serve hot.

(4 servings)   42 cal. per serving.

HARVARD BEETS

3 c. sliced beets (cooked)
2 t. dietary sweetener
1 T. cornstarch
1/2 c. beet juice
1/2 c. cider vinegar

Combine sweetener, cornstarch, beet juice. Add vinegar.
Bring to a boil slowly, stirring constantly until sauce has thickened. Add beets and allow to simmer until beets are heated through.

Season to taste with a dietary salt substitute.
(6 servings)   50 cal. per serving.

VEGETABLE STEW (Ratatouille)

1 sm. eggplant, diced
3 med. tomatoes, quartered
2 med. onions, chopped
3 sm. zucchini, sliced
2 green peppers, chopped
1 clove garlic, minced
3 T. chopped parsley
2 T. corn-oil margarine
pepper to taste

Sauté vegetables in corn-oil margarine until soft. Do not brown. Stir in minced garlic. Add chopped parsley. Add pepper and dietary salt substitute to taste.

(Seasoned dietary salt is especially good.)
(6 servings)   90 cal. per serving.

BAKED MUSHROOMS

8 large mushrooms
1 t. corn oil
1/2 onion, chopped fine
2 T. minced green pepper
1/8 lb. very lean ground round steak
2 T. tomato juice
lemon juice

Clean and dry mushrooms. Mince the stems, leaving the caps whole. Sauté the chopped mushroom stems, onion, and green pepper until tender. Stir in ground meat and cook until meat loses its red color. Remove from heat and stir in tomato juice and a few drops of lemon juice. Fill mushroom caps with this mixture. Bake, filled side up, at 350° for 20 minutes. Use diet salt substitute to taste.

(4 servings)   20 cal. per mushroom.

Spinach Casserole

1 c. cooked spinach (well drained)	40 cal.
1/2 c. cottage cheese	100 cal.
1/2 small tomato (garnish)	10 cal.
Total	150 cal.

Baked Potato-1 portion

1/2 baked potato	50 cal.
1/4 c. cottage cheese	50 cal.
few chives	0 cal.
Total	100 cal.

Basic Eggplant

Peel and dice 1 large eggplant	50 cal.
1/2 large onion	25 cal.
1/2 green pepper (diced)	9 cal.
3 diced garlic cloves	6 cal.
Sweetener to taste	0 cal.
1 c. Basic Tomato Sauce	100 cal.
Total	190 cal.

Skillet Pepper and Tomatoes

2 green peppers
3 med. tomatoes
1 T. margarine
1 1/2 c. sliced onions
1/4 t. pepper
1/4 t. oregano
garlic powder to taste

Cut peppers into thin strips. Cut tomatoes into eighths (do not peel; the skin is excellent roughage).

Melt the margarine in a nonstick skillet over low heat. Add onion and sauté until tender. Add peppers, tomatoes, and seasonings. Cover skillet and simmer for 10 minutes.

(6 servings)   43 cal. per serving.

Carbohydrate 8 gm. Protein 2 gm. Fat negligible.

Red Cabbage and Applesauce

1 lb. red cabbage
1/2 c. sliced onion
2 c. unsweetened applesauce
1/4 t. black pepper
1 T. caraway seeds

Shred cabbage and combine with rest of ingredients. Cover pot and simmer for 30 to 40 minutes, stirring occasionally. Season with diet salt.

(6 servings)   58 cal. per serving.

Carbohydrate 14.8 gm. Protein 1.6 gm. Fat 0.

Desserts

Citrus Sauce Compote

3 oranges
3 t. orange peel, grated
1/2 c. water
1/4 t. vanilla extract
1/8 t. ground cloves
sugar substitute equal to 1 T. sugar

Finely grate the orange peel, being careful to use only the orange-colored part. Peel and dice the oranges over a bowl to catch the juice. Pour the juice into a saucepan. Add the water, vanilla, and ground cloves. Bring to a boil, and boil for three minutes. Add the diced oranges and simmer for 10 more minutes. Cool and refrigerate. When cold, add sugar substitute and mix well. Excellent served chilled as a light dessert. Try it warmed on broiled chicken.

(4 servings)   40 cal. per serving.

PARTY PEARS

8 ripe, firm pears (Bartlett are best)
2 cups water
2 t. vanilla extract
1 t. rum extract
sugar substitute equal to 2/3 c. sugar
1/2 t. cinnamon
4 drops red food coloring

Cut pears in half. Peel and core carefully. Put vanilla, rum extract, sugar substitute, cinnamon, and red coloring in a saucepan and bring to a slow boil. Place the pears in simmering water and cook, turning frequently, about 10 minutes, until easily pierced with a fork but not soft.

DIET BAKED APPLES

Place apples in baking dish. Sprinkle with cinnamon. Pour one can of diet soda (any flavor*) over them. Bake at 350° F. until soft (about 30 minutes). Turn apples once during baking.

* Diet lemon and diet ginger ale are very good. If not sweet enough, add more sugar substitute after cooking.

FROZEN BANANAS

Place bananas, with skin intact, in freezer. Tastes like banana ice cream when frozen. The skin will turn very dark, but the flesh will stay the natural color.

DIET APPLE PIE

4 apples	300 cal.
12 oz. lemon diet soda	0 cal.
2 pks. unflavored gelatin	56 cal.
2 pks. Sweet 'n Low	0 cal.
1/3 c. dry skim milk	90 cal.
cinnamon	

Peel and core apples. Arrange in baking dish. Soak gelatin in diet soda. Add Sweet 'n Low; dissolve. Pour over apples in pie pan. Sprinkle with skim-milk powder.

Dust with cinnamon or apple-pie spice. Bake at 350 degrees for 45 minutes. Cool. Chill in refrigerator.

(8 servings)   56 cal. per serving.

SOMETHING WITH NOTHING (or a Smashing Spoof)

1 env. unflav. gelatin
1/4 c. cold water
3/4 c. boiling water
sugar substitute equal to 1 T. sugar
1/4 t. vanilla extract
1 t. strawberry extract
1 c. cold water
mint sprigs

Put the gelatin in a cup and soften with 1/4 c. cold water. Add boiling water and stir until the gelatin is completely dissolved. Add the sugar substitute and extracts. Refrigerate until very firm.

When mixture is firm, put into a blender. Add 1 c. cold water and blend at high speed until frothy. Pour into sherbet glasses and garnish with mint sprigs!

Variations: Instead of strawberry extract, any extract you wish may be substituted. For example:

1/2 t. vanilla extract plus 1/2 t. rum extract. Garnish with nutmeg.

1/2 t. vanilla extract plus 1/2 t. orange extract. Garnish with orange peel.

1/2 t. vanilla extract plus 1 T. grated lemon peel. Garnish with lemon twist.

2 t. instant coffee plus 1/4 t. cinnamon. Garnish with a small piece of cinnamon stick and a touch of Whipped Milk Topping.

1/4 t. vanilla extract plus 1/2 t. coconut extract. Garnish with crushed pineapple.

1/2 t. vanilla extract plus 1/2 t. almond extract. Garnish with Whipped

Milk Topping or pour a little milk over the top and sprinkle with a few raisins.

Approx. 5 calories per serving.

POPPY-SEED CAKE

1/2 c. poppy seeds
1 c. skim milk
21/4 c. flour
11/2 c. sugar
6 t. low-sodium baking powder
1/2 c. unsalted margarine
11/4 t. vanilla
4 egg whites, beaten

Soak poppy seeds in skim milk. Mix dry ingredients. Add margarine, poppy-seed/milk mixture, and vanilla. Mix on medium speed for 2 minutes. Fold in egg whites. Pour into 13 × 9 × 2 baking pan; bake in preheated 350-degree-F oven for 30 minutes or until done. Cut in 117 1-inch squares; 110 calories per square.

Relishes, Sauces and Toppings

BASIC TOMATO SAUCE

1 large onion	50 cal.
1 large green pepper	20 cal.
6 tomatoes (peeled)	120 cal.
3 cloves garlic	6 cal.
ground black pepper	0 cal.
oregano	0 cal.
basil	0 cal.
Total	196 cal.

Sweetener to taste. Put in pot, add 2 tablespoons water. Cover and simmer until well done.

(Approx. 4 servings)   Approx. 50 cal. per serving.

DIET COCKTAIL SAUCE FOR FISH

2 T. diet catsup
1/2 t. prepared horseradish

(1 serving)   20 cal. per serving.

JELLED MILK

1 env. unflav. gelatin
1/4 c. water
1 c. milk (nonfat, low-fat, whole, or
buttermilk may be used)

Put the water in a small saucepan. Sprinkle the gelatin on the top and allow it to soften. Place the saucepan on low heat, stirring constantly until the gelatin is completely dissolved. Do not allow it to come to a boil.

Slowly pour the milk into the gelatin, stirring as you do.

Place the gelatin-milk mixture in the refrigerator. When it is jelled it is ready to use as Jelled Milk for many recipes.

WHIPPED MILK TOPPING

1 c. Jelled Milk
1 c. cold milk (skim)
sugar substitute equal to 1 T. sugar
1/2 t. vanilla (or any extract you
like)

Put all ingredients in the blender and blend on high speed until frothy. Cover and store in the refrigerator.

This topping is fabulous on fresh or poached fruit.

Whipped Buttermilk Topping

Use same procedure and ingredients as for Whipped Milk Topping, but substitute whipped buttermilk for the whipped milk and cold buttermilk for the cold milk. I like to add more vanilla, too, perhaps a whole teaspoon. I like this topping best with baked apples, pineapple, and fresh oranges. It is also a good dressing on fruit salads.

1/4 c. = 20 cal.

Fresh Cranberry Relish

1 lb. (4 c.) fresh cranberries
2 sm. oranges
sugar substitute equal to 1 c. sugar

Wash oranges well and grate 2 tablespoons of the peel. Be careful to grate only the orange-colored part of the peel.

Peel the oranges and cut them in pieces, removing seeds and connecting membranes. Put them in the blender with the sugar substitute and grated peel. Mix well. Add the cranberries, a few at a time, until all of the berries have been blended into the relish. Don't blend it too fine, as you want a fairly coarse relish.

Make this several days before Thanksgiving or whenever you plan to serve it. It is much better after sitting in the refrigerator for three or four days.

(Makes 4 cups)   10 cal. per 1/2-cup serving.

Strawberry Jam

2 c. fresh strawberries (or fresh-
   frozen without sugar)
1 t. lemon juice
1 t. unflav. gelatin
sugar substitute equal to 2 T. sugar

Put the strawberries, whole, in a covered saucepan. Cook, covered, over very low heat without water for about 10 minutes. Remove the lid and bring the juice to the boiling point. Boil for 1 minute and remove from heat. Soften the gelatin in the lemon juice. Pour some of the hot juice from the strawberries into the gelatin mix, and then add to the strawberries. Allow to cool to room temperature. Add sugar substitute and refrigerate.

Variations: You can use this same recipe for any fresh-fruit jam. However, I think it is best for peaches, pineapple,* and berries of all types.

* Use canned pineapple.

Stress, Personality, and Heart Disease

The image of the ambitious, hard-driving, coronary-prone man-on-the-rise is a popular one in the public mind. So is the notion that the stress of modern living causes heart attacks. As early as 1897, Sir William Osler—often considered the father of modern medicine—wrote: "In the worry and strain of modern life, arterial degeneration is not only very common, but develops often at a relatively early age. For this I believe that the high pressure at which men live and the habit of working the machine to its maximum capacity, are responsible rather than excesses in eating and drinking. . . ."

In agreement with Dr. Osler, the general public has long associated the heart with a variety of emotional and physical responses: "She died of a broken heart," "He just didn't have the heart to do it," "My heart leapt with joy when I saw him," are common examples of how we relate the heart to mind and body. By the same token, we often search for an emotional or personality factor to explain heart disease: "He worked himself into a heart attack," or "His rage finally got the best of him and he keeled over with a heart attack." But the medical community has been slow to agree, and it has been only in the past few years that large numbers of doctors and researchers have accepted the idea that stress and personality may be important cardiovascular risk factors. In 1954, for example, Dr. W. M. Arnott summed up the opinion of many physicians and researchers of thirty years ago when he wrote in the *British Medical Journal:* "So far as I can see, this hypothesis [i.e., the possible relationship of nervous stress and strain to coronary artery disease] has no scientifically credible basis whatsoever—in fact most of the evidence adduced in its support is dubious and much of it absurd."

Once again the tide of medical opinion is turning, and today stress and the way we respond to it are thought to be among the life-style factors that may increase the risk of a heart attack. The shift began in the nineteen sixties and seventies, as results of large-scale epidemiologic studies confirmed the public suspicion that certain personality traits were strongly correlated with an increased incidence of heart disease. Although the evidence was largely circumstantial, it was based on the same kind of statistical findings linking heart disease to smoking, obesity, and other life-style factors. For example, Thomas Holmes and Richard Rahe, two researchers at the University of Washington, studied the relationship between a number of stressful life changes and disease in more than five thousand people. They identified more than forty life events, ranging from the death of a spouse and divorce to holidays and minor scrapes with the law, that seemed to increase the chance of falling ill. The more upsetting the event the greater the likelihood of illness. And if several changes occurred in quick succession, the likelihood increased even more. The illnesses ranged from catching a cold to heart attacks and cancer. (See the accompanying Social Readjustment Rating Scale, pages 163–64.)

But being subjected to stress is not the only factor. Indeed, given the pace of modern life, stress is almost impossible to avoid. How we cope with the stress is also thought to be important, and this is where our individual personalities come in. Much of the current interest in the possible role of personality and heart disease can be traced to two San Francisco cardiologists and researchers, Drs. Meyer Friedman and Ray Rosenman. In the mid-1950s, they began their famous Type-A-personality studies. In his book *Pathogenesis of Coronary Artery Disease,* Dr. Friedman recalls: "It was approximately at the same time [1955] that we were perusing the available literature concerning cholesterol metabolism and heart disease . . . that we began to observe the presence of certain traits in almost every one of our middle-aged and younger coronary patients. . . . Exactly why it took us more than a decade to observe traits which now almost 'shout' at us, we don't know."

What were these characteristic traits? Drs. Friedman and Rosenman defined them as excessive drive and ambition to succeed; aggressive, competitive, hostile feelings toward others; a harrowing sense of time urgency; difficulty in adapting to change—hallmarks of Type A personality.

An urgency about time is one of the chief Type A characteristics. The Type A person always seems to be in a hurry, and cannot tolerate the idea of wasting time or being late. His or her talk is punctuated with such statements as: "I don't know where the time goes" or "There are not enough hours in the day to get everything done." Type A's walk, talk, and eat fast, and are quick to show impatience with those who are slower-paced. They will finish sentences for people who speak slowly, and constantly prod others to "hurry up."

In the extreme, the Type A is always ready to react with maximum effort, even if the situation does not call for such a response. The appropriate level of response for any given task is defined by the Yerkes-Dodson Law, which holds that there is an optimal level of arousal, or stress, at which performance will be most effective. This level is defined by the complexity of the task to be performed: a simple task requires only moderate stress, while a more complex one involves a greater level of arousal to get the job done. In short, a certain degree of stress is necessary if we are to perform effectively. We need to feel we are in control of the situation and can meet its demands. But, beyond a certain optimal level, stress can have a disruptive effect on the entire body and we are no longer in control. This can lead to negative feelings and actually cause a decline in ability to perform. In this respect, Type A's seem to operate on a short fuse, with frequent outbursts of anger or hostility. In contrast, the Type B person in the same situation is slower to react. In general, Type B's are not as hard-driving or anxious to succeed, and not as pressured by time. Type B's are easygoing, and generally trusting of others.

ARE YOU A TYPE A?

Some studies have found that at least 50 percent, and perhaps as many as 75 percent, of all American adults are Type A. What's more, the behavior pattern appears early in life: studies have found that as early as age eleven or twelve, the familiar traits appear. Of course, we live in a highly competitive, success-oriented society, in which many of the characteristics of Type A behavior are considered the norm, the necessary ingredients of success. Indeed, we often worry about a youngster who is not motivated to give his or her all. It is not surprising, then, that many Type A's do not recognize themselves as such. While many people readily recognize and admit to the more socially acceptable Type A traits—assertiveness, strength, self-confidence, ambition, persistence, and being fast-paced, outgoing, and talkative— the more negative ones—hostility, irritability, impulsiveness, restlessness, bossiness, self-centeredness, and stubbornness—are often denied by those whose personality tests indicate these traits. Indeed, one of the problems faced by doctors has been to identify true Type A's and then to zero in on those Type A traits that seem to be more harmful than others. A number of tests, usually involving questionnaires designed to detect certain personality traits, have been developed in recent years; these are now widely used to assess behavior types. Typical questions might include:

1. Do you have difficulty in finding time to shop or visit friends?
2. Do you find yourself finishing sentences for slow talkers?
3. How do you react if you have to wait in line at the bank or a store?

4. How seriously do you take your work?
5. Are you quick-tempered or easygoing?
6. Do you feel compelled to win, even if your opponent is a child or other easy match?
7. Do you often bring work home?
8. Do you often set deadlines for yourself?
9. Do you always seem to be in a hurry?
10. Do you feel you can trust most people?
11. Are you able to relax at home or when on vacation? Or do you find yourself thinking about work and calling in daily?
12. Do you usually assume a leadership role in any group activity?

As noted earlier, many of the Type A personality traits are considered highly desirable in our success-oriented society. And many Type A's have no desire to change: They like taking charge and being constantly on the go. Is there a happy medium that will allow people to drive for success and still avoid the possible adverse effects on their health? In an effort to further define the personality traits that may be the most closely linked to heart disease, researchers at Duke University and a number of other centers have conducted studies comparing various aspects of behavior with health. While the evidence is far from conclusive, these studies seem to indicate that feelings of hostility may be among the most damaging.

One of these studies—a joint effort of researchers at Duke University Medical Center and the University of North Carolina—followed a group of 255 physicians for twenty-five years. While still in medical school, the participants had taken personality tests that separated the Type A's from the Type B's. In this particular analysis, the researchers looked specifically at the hostility scores, to see if those with the most pronounced feelings of hostility—for example, feelings of distrust and isolation—had a higher incidence of heart disease. Even when other risk factors, such as smoking, elevated cholesterol, age, and a family history of heart disease were accounted for, they found that among the men who were still living, those whose hostility scores were above the median had an almost sixfold higher incidence of coronary events as compared to those whose scores were below the median.

When examining the backgrounds of those who died in the twenty-five years since completing medical school, the researchers found a striking, but unexpected, relationship between the hostility scores and death from all causes. There had been nineteen deaths among the 255 physicians: four from heart attacks, two from other cardiovascular problems, four from cancer, eight from accidents or suicide, and one from gastrointestinal disease. Of these, only three (whose causes of death were heart attack, cancer, and an accident) had hostility scores below the median. The chance of death was more than six times greater for the more hostile group. In short, not only were the hostility scores good predictors for death from a heart attack; they also pointed to those at risk of premature death from other causes.

This study seems to confirm results of other research at Duke and elsewhere. At least four studies, in which patients undergoing examination of their coronary arteries (coronary arteriography) were also subjected to personality testing, have found that patients in the Type A group also have the most severe coronary disease. In a Duke University Medical Center study, for example, personality tests were administered to 424 patients undergoing coronary arteriography because of suspected coronary heart disease. The research team, led by Drs. James A. Blumenthal and Redford B. Williams, found that the patients with the most severe disease also had the highest hostility scores—a finding that applied to both men and women. (See graph, page 165.)

A long-term study of 1,877 men employed by Western Electric in Chicago also found their hostility scores correlated with coronary events. And again the men with the higher hostility scores had a higher overall death rate than their less hostile colleagues. In fact, those in the group with the highest hostility scores had a 42 percent increase in the risk of death over the next twenty years over those with the lowest scores.

So far, researchers have not come up with an explanation of why feelings of hostility should increase the risk of a heart attack and death from other causes. They point, however, to other studies that have found people who lack adequate social support—divorced or unmarried men, immigrants cut off from family and cultural tradition, for example—also have a higher risk of heart attacks and a higher overall mortality rate. Two researchers who have studied hostility and heart disease—Drs. W. W. Cook and D. M. Medley—have noted that since a person with deep feelings of hostility "has little confidence in his fellow man and sees people as dishonest, unsocial, immoral, ugly and mean," it is not unreasonable to speculate that he also lacks meaningful social supports. Whether or not there is, indeed, a connection between this and heart disease will require additional study to confirm; in the meantime, it seems clear that feelings of hostility are unhealthful and, over a period of years, greatly increase the chances of death, not only from heart attacks but from other causes as well.

BIOCHEMISTRY OF TYPE A'S

If we accept the thesis that personality factors and the way we respond to stress are related to heart disease, the next logical step is to determine the mechanisms by which behavior affects the body.

To try to come up with the answers, researchers are now looking at the ways in which we react to stress, which ranges from the pressures of everyday living to sudden, unexpected danger. Our reaction to stress, especially when danger is involved, is often referred to as the "fight-or-flight response." It is an almost automatic reaction, characterized by a quickened heart rate, increased blood pressure, tensed muscles, and a heightened awareness—all appropriate automatic reactions that can be life-saving in certain situations, because they give us the extra strength or speed to get out of difficult situations. When translated to our everyday lives, this hyperresponse may be appropriate in making important business decisions, avoiding a traffic accident, or rescuing a child from a dangerous situation. But such a response is not necessary or appropriate in performing routine tasks or making ordinary, day-to-day decisions. A recent study by Duke researchers has found, however, that Type A's tend to overreact to almost any challenge, no matter how routine.

In this study, twenty-four Type A's and seventeen Type B's were enlisted to participate in a verbal problem-solving experiment. Some of the participants were offered small monetary rewards as an added incentive. As might be expected, the Type A's answered more questions more quickly than the Type B's, particularly when the cash incentives were added. During all phases of the tests, blood pressure, heart rate, and other cardiovascular responses of all the participants were measured, and here the researchers noted some marked differences between the Type A's and the Type B's. No cardiovascular changes occurred in the Type B's until the cash incentives were offered; then their heart rates and blood pressures went up and the blood vessels that supply the skeletal muscles became wider (vasodilation). In contrast, the Type A's showed these changes in all problem-solving situations; the addition of cash incentives made little or no difference. In other words, Type A's tend to overreact even when there is no incentive to do so, while Type B's are more likely to respond according to the task at hand and the stakes involved.

This tendency of Type A's to overreact appears to affect the entire body. Studies have found that Type A hyperresponders have elevated levels of catecholamines—naturally occurring chemicals that include dopamine and norepinephrine. These chemicals stimulate the sympathetic nervous **system,** which, among other things, controls the size of blood vessels, which in turns affects blood pressure. Type A's also tend to have higher levels of certain sex hormones—a consistent factor that a group of Columbia University researchers have found in heart-attack patients.

Exactly how these biochemical changes might trigger heart disease is unknown, but one popular theory goes like this: As we have seen, three basic events are involved in the development of atherosclerosis: (1) the overgrowth (proliferation) of the smooth-muscle cells that line the arteries; (2) the buildup of cholesterol and other fatty deposits along the arterial walls; and (3) the accumulation of other substances, such as collagen and elastic fibers, to form the atherosclerotic plaque (atheromas). Researchers theorize that the process is set in motion by some sort of injury to the tissue that lines the arterial walls (the endothelium). It is conceivable that the frequent surges of norepinephrine and other blood chemicals experienced by Type A's, and the resultant increased stress and turbulence seen in the cardiovascular system, cause this initial injury to the artery walls, thereby initiating the atherosclerosis. Recent studies involving laboratory animals indicate that daily exposure to stress does result in the buildup of fatty deposits in the artery walls, and laboratory animals exposed to stress have a higher death rate from both heart disease and cancer. This does not mean, of course, that the same applies to humans, but it is one more piece of evidence pointing to a link between behavior and heart disease.

ALTERING TYPE A BEHAVIOR

If we accept the idea that Type A behavior increases the risk of a heart attack, then it would seem logical that changing the behavior is a sound approach to preventing heart disease. Indeed, recent studies at Duke indicate that modifying Type A behavior among heart-attack patients, along with stopping smoking, are the only two life-style modifications that help prevent subsequent heart attacks. (This does not include physiological actions, such as taking drugs to stabilize heart rhythm or undergoing coronary bypass surgery.) Unfortunately, many Type A's, as noted earlier, are either unaware of their potentially harmful behavior or are reluctant to change. They enjoy their fast-paced, hyper lives and credit their success to their excessive drive.

The key, then, is to modify the more destructive aspects of their behavior —such as their inappropriate overreaction to any problem or excessive feelings of hostility and anger—while preserving the positive attributes. DUPAC offers two approaches that seem to work for most Type A participants. One involves physical activity—the cornerstone of DUPAC—and the other involves behavior-modification training using such techniques as psychological counseling, biofeedback, and relaxation training.

THE ROLE OF EXERCISE

As noted in earlier chapters, a number of studies have equated increased physical activity with a lowered risk of heart attacks and other manifestations of coronary heart disease. The reasons for this are unknown, but a number of theories have been advanced, and one hypothesis involves the modification of Type A behavior as a result of regular exercise. To investigate this theory, a group of Duke researchers—Drs. James A. Blumenthal, R. Sanders Williams, Redford B. Williams, Jr., and Andrew G. Wallace—enlisted a group of forty-six healthy volunteers to study the effects of fitness training on behavior. The participants—twenty men and twenty-six women—were subjected to a number of medical and psychological tests before embarking on a ten-week fitness program. All were judged free of heart disease after physical examination and an exercise stress test. The psychological testing found that twenty-one were Type A and twenty-five were Type B.

The fitness program consisted of three 40- to 55-minute sessions a week, with each session providing 10 minutes of warm-up exercises followed by 30 to 45 minutes of walking or jogging. After the ten weeks, the participants repeated the tests performed at the beginning of the program. As might be expected, the researchers found a marked improvement in physical condition after the training program, as documented in increased endurance during the treadmill stress test.

In addition, several cardiovascular risk factors were altered for both the Type A's and the Type B's. Although there was no change in total blood cholesterol, there was a significant increase in HDL cholesterol. There was also a significant drop in weight, particularly among the Type A's. Blood pressure was also lowered for both groups.

As for the psychological benefits, the study documented for the first time that a fitness program can achieve significant reductions in the degree of Type A behavior. The Type A's were not transformed into Type B's—this was not the goal. But excessive Type A behavior was measurably reduced. Although the researchers do not know the reason for this moderation in Type A behavior, they offer several possibilities. For example, ". . . it is possible that the exercise program encouraged [the study] subjects to reorder their priorities and make significant alterations in their life-styles. Social interactions may also have had a therapeutic effect."

The researchers emphasize that although this study does not conclusively prove that exercise will actually reduce the possibility of future heart attacks, the findings do suggest a "potential usefulness of this inexpensive, cost-effective program for altering the risk profile of Type A subjects."

A subsequent study further documents the psychological benefits of exercise. This study involved two groups: eleven women and five men, twenty-five to sixty-one years old, who signed up for a ten-week fitness program, and a matched control group who went about their normal routines without any exercise conditioning. Again, all the participants underwent physical and psychological testing both before and after the fitness program, which was similar to the one followed in the first study.

Pretesting found no significant differences between the two groups in the six areas being measured: tension, depression, anxiety, vigor, fatigue, and confusion. Several important differences emerged in the post-testing, however. Two thirds of the exercise group felt that their general health was improved at the end of the ten weeks, and 61 percent felt an enhanced sense of personal achievement. In contrast, only 16 percent of the sedentary (control) group felt that their health had improved, and 27 percent reported an enhanced sense of achievement, which is not considered statistically significant.

Anxiety and depression were significantly reduced in the exercise group, and unchanged or even worsened among the controls. Similarly, the exercise group experienced reduced tension, confusion, and fatigue, and increased vigor, while the scores for these traits remained unchanged for the controls. In summarizing the importance of these findings, the Duke researchers noted that "while the psychological benefits of physical exercise have been propagandized in the popular press, there has been a paucity of objective evidence for this assertion. The major finding of this study is the significant improvement in the overall psychological functioning of subjects participating in a brief, structured exercise program. In virtually every comparison, the exercise group changed in the desired direction, while the control group remained the same or actually got worse." Although this study did not differentiate between Type A's and Type B's, it did demonstrate that exercise helped reduce anxiety and tension—two traits common to Type A behavior—in all participants.

LEARNING HOW TO COPE WITH STRESS

Upon enrolling in DUPAC, participants are seen by one of the staff psychologists. About one third are found to be suffering from anxiety or depression—common disorders among people who have had heart attacks or other cardiovascular symptoms. These disorders are treated in the traditional manner, usually by psychoanalysis or group therapy.

Personality type is also assessed, with particular attention paid to identifying Type A characteristics. Those who have difficulty in coping with stress or are unable to relax or control anger and hostility or other negative feelings, are taught how to modify their behavior. This involves behavioral training aimed at providing coping techniques. Learning how to recognize and plan for stressful situations, as well as being able to physically relax, are the key elements.

The relaxation exercises taught to DUPAC patients are modeled on the progressive muscle-relaxation training developed by Dr. Edmund Jacobson at Harvard University nearly fifty years ago. Dr. Jacobson's stress studies found that emotional tension shortens muscle fibers and that this tension can be relieved by progressively relaxing muscles throughout the body. DUPAC's Dr. Blumenthal recommends that the following relaxation exercises be practiced twice a day until they are mastered. "At first," he says, "they will take about thirty minutes of practice, but as you master the technique, the time required will become progressively shorter." In fact, one DUPAC patient who participated in the behavior-modification program says, "I can now shut my office door and be fully relaxed in about fifteen or twenty minutes, and feel like I've just wakened from a good night's sleep. I'm ready to put in another three or four productive hours, instead of feeling tense and dragged out."

HOW TO RELAX

Here are the relaxation exercises recommended by Dr. Blumenthal, as adapted from a DUPAC patient-education booklet.

1. Get as comfortable as possible. Loosen tight clothing. Legs should not be crossed. Take a deep breath and let it out slowly.

2. Raise your arms and extend them out in front of you. Make fists with both hands as hard as you can. Note the uncomfortable tension in your hands and fingers. Hold the tension for five seconds, then let the tension out halfway and hold for an additional five seconds. Notice the decrease in tension, but also concentrate on the tension that is still present. Then let your hands relax completely. Notice how the tension and discomfort drain from your hands and are replaced by sensations of comfort and relaxation. Focus on the contrast between the tension you

created and the contrasting state of relaxation you now feel. Concentrate on relaxing your hands completely for fifteen seconds.

3. Tense your bicepses hard for five seconds by bending your arms at the elbows. Again, focus on the feeling of tension. Then let the tension out halfway for an additional five seconds, and focus on the tension that remains. Now relax your upper arms completely for fifteen seconds and focus carefully on the developing sense of relaxation.

4. Bend your hands at the wrist, extending your fingers upward as far as possible. Hold the tension for five seconds, then let the tension out halfway for an additional five seconds. Now relax the muscles completely and concentrate on the relaxation until they are completely loose.

5. Now tense your neck muscles by bringing your head forward until your chin digs into your chest. Hold for five seconds, release the tension halfway for another five seconds, and then relax your neck completely. Allow your head to hang comfortably while you focus on the relaxation developing in your neck muscles.

6. Tense your upper shoulders by shrugging them: try to touch your shoulders to your ears. Let the tension out halfway and hold for five seconds, and then relax completely. Let your shoulders drop down and get completely relaxed.

7. Push your shoulders back as far as possible so as to tense your back muscles. Let the tension out halfway after five seconds, and then relax your back and shoulder muscles completely. Focus on the spreading relaxation until they are totally relaxed.

8. Now move to the muscles of your face. First, wrinkle your forehead as hard as possible. Hold the tension for five seconds, then release halfway for another five seconds, and then relax your scalp and forehead completely, as always focusing on the developing feeling of relaxation and contrasting it with the tension that existed earlier.

9. With your eyes closed, squint as hard as you can. Hold the tension for five seconds, then release it halfway for an additional five seconds. Then relax your eyes completely. Focus on the relaxation developing in your eyes and also concentrate on relaxing your other facial muscles.

10. Tense your tongue by pushing it into the roof of your mouth as hard as possible. Hold for five seconds, then let the tension out halfway and hold for an additional five seconds. Then relax your tongue completely, focusing on completely relaxing the muscles of your neck, jaw, and tongue.

11. Take a deep breath and hold it, expanding your chest as much as possible. Now relax: exhale and continue breathing as you were. Notice

that your breathing is getting slower and more regular as you get more relaxed.

12. Tense your stomach muscles as hard as possible for five seconds and concentrate on the tension. Then let the tension out halfway for an additional five seconds before relaxing your stomach muscles completely. Focus on the spreading relaxation until your stomach muscles are completely relaxed.

13. Tense your buttock muscles hard for five seconds, then let the tension out halfway for another five seconds. Finally, relax your buttocks completely and focus on the sensations of heaviness and relaxation. Concentrate on also relaxing the muscle groups you have already dealt with.

14. Extend your legs and raise them approximately six inches above the floor and tense your thigh muscles. Hold the tension for five seconds, let it out halfway for an additional five seconds, and then relax your thighs completely.

15. Bend your feet at the ankles, extending your toes upward toward your head. Feel the tension in your feet and calves. Let it out halfway for an additional five seconds, and then relax your feet and calves completely for fifteen seconds.

16. With your feet on the floor and your legs relaxed, dig the toes of your feet in the bottom of your shoes. After five seconds, relax the toes halfway and hold the reduced tension for an additional five seconds. Then relax your toes completely and focus on the relaxation spreading into the toes. Continue relaxing your toes for fifteen seconds. Concentrate on totally relaxing your feet, calves, and thighs for thirty seconds.

17. Deep breathing is one of the most important elements of the relaxation response, since one can bring forth a feeling of relaxation by correct breathing. Take a series of short inhalations, about one per second, until the lungs are filled. Hold for about five seconds, then exhale slowly for about ten seconds while thinking silently to yourself the word "relax" or the word "calm." Picture the word to yourself as you slowly let out your breath. Repeat the process at least five times, each time attempting to deepen the state of relaxation you are experiencing. Continue to relax for ten minutes. When you finish, open your eyes and sit quietly for a few more minutes. By now, you should feel alert and refreshed.

For those who find it difficult to learn progressive relaxation, biofeedback training is a useful tool. During biofeedback training, a person learns how to control certain body responses and functions, including some that are normally involuntary, such as heart rate and blood pressure. DUPAC participants learn the basic techniques by listening to an audio cassette outlining the progressive relaxation exercises. The biofeedback training sessions take place in a quiet, darkened room. Sensors are attached to the body to measure heart rate, blood pressure, muscle tension, and other body functions. An inappropriate response—for example, one in which the blood pressure, heart rate, and muscle tension increase—is signaled by a beeping noise or a light. The task is to control the body to stop the signal. After a few sessions, in the words of a long-time DUPAC participant, Wendall Austin, "progressive relaxation becomes second nature to your mind and body, even in acutely stressful experiences."

Other useful coping techniques include the ability to recognize stressful situations and plan accordingly. "For example," says Dr. Blumenthal, "learning how to prepare for a public speech is helpful in reducing the stress involved in giving talks before an audience."

How we look at ourselves is yet another determinant in how well we cope with stress. Dr. Blumenthal explains: "An individual who responds to his boss's criticism by telling himself that he's worthless or incompetent will have a very different physical and emotional reaction than the individual who tells himself, 'So I'm having an off day. I'll learn from my mistake and do better next time.'"

Learning how to recognize stress and judging your tension levels in various situations is another useful tool in stress management. "Keep a daily diary in which you note your experience of stress during the week," Dr. Blumenthal urges. "The goal of successful stress management is to reduce or eliminate unpleasant feelings and to substitute more pleasant and adaptive responses." One way you may learn to become more aware of your tension level is to regularly rate your tension levels on a scale of one to ten throughout the day, with one representing total relaxation and ten your highest level of tension. Pay particular attention to your level of muscle tension. If you tense up while waiting in line or for a traffic light, practice some of the muscle-relaxation techniques outlined earlier. Avoiding situations that produce tension is still another effective coping technique. If you can't stand waiting in line at the bank or post office, time your trips to such places to avoid lines.

SUMMING UP

It is increasingly clear that stress and our reaction to it has a profound effect upon our overall health. A growing number of physicians and heart researchers feel that Type A personality traits, particularly excessive feelings of hostility, are a risk factor for coronary disease. Therefore, it is important to recognize these detrimental personality traits in ourselves and take steps to modify them. This does not mean that we should try to transform Type A's into Type B's; instead, we should look for those traits that are considered the most excessive and harmful and concentrate on changing them. Duke researchers have identified two important avenues for altering Type A behavior: exercise training and behavior modification. The latter may involve psychological counseling, group therapy, or relaxation training that may include biofeedback training. Learning to control stress and modify destructive personality traits should not be construed as a cure for heart disease. But learning to cope and overcoming feelings of frustration and tension will certainly make life more enjoyable, and very likely, healthier as well.

There is mounting evidence that altering Type A behavior may have benefits that go beyond reducing the risk of heart disease. Studies at Duke and elsewhere have found that Type A's—particularly those who are overly hostile—have a higher rate of premature death from all causes. And, of course, there are those intangible rewards of well-being and an enhanced enjoyment of life that come with controlling some of the more negative aspects of Type A behavior.

Table 1. Adjectives Rated as Characteristic or Uncharacteristic of Type A Individuals

% ENDORSING	CHARACTERISTIC	UNCHARACTERISTIC
100	Aggressive, hurried	Easygoing
90	Active, alert, ambitious, assertive, dominant, energetic, hostile, impatient, irritable, quick	Calm, relaxed
80	Determined, forceful, impulsive, restless	Mild, patient, slow, unambitious
70	Argumentative, bossy, excitable, industrious, persistent, tense	Leisurely, quiet, reflective, unexcitable

60	Confident, demanding, enterprising, hasty, opinionated, outspoken, self-centered, strong	Retiring, silent, submissive, weak
50	Enthusiastic, hardheaded, headstrong, individualistic, loud, masculine, persevering, self-confident, stubborn	Apathetic, cautious, contented, dreamy, feminine, gentle, lazy, meek, shy, timid, withdrawn

Table 2. Hostility Scale of Items Endorsed by at Least a 20% Greater Proportion of Patients Scoring 11–15 on the Total Hostility Scale, Compared to Patients Scoring 10 or Less

DIFFERENCE IN PROPORTION ENDORSING ITEM (%)	CONTENT OF ITEM
35	I have often met people who were supposed to be experts who were no better than I.
30	When a man is with a woman, he is usually thinking about things related to her sex.
25	I would certainly enjoy beating a crook at his own game.
24	I have at times had to be rough with people who were rude or annoying.
24	I do not try to cover up my poor opinion or pity of a person so that he won't know how I feel.

| 22 | I have frequently worked under people who seem to have things arranged so that they get credit for good work but are able to pass off mistakes onto those under them. |

| 22 | I have often had to take orders from someone who did not know as much as I did. |

| 20 | Some of my family have habits that bother and annoy me very much. |

| 20 | A large number of people are guilty of bad sexual conduct. |

Type A Self-Test

SPECIAL INSTRUCTIONS

You will be shown a number of adjectives. We would like you to use these words to describe yourself by indicating, on a scale of 1 to 7, how true of *you* these various characteristics are. Please give your own opinion of yourself. If you are not sure, put down the number that comes closest to what you think best describes you. Do not leave any blank spaces if you can avoid it.

Example: Sly
Make a 1 if it is *never or almost never true* that you are sly.
Mark a 2 if it is *usually not true* that you are sly.
Mark a 3 if it is *sometimes but infrequently true* that you are sly.
Mark a 4 if it is *occasionally true* that you are sly.
Mark a 5 if it is *often true* that you are sly.
Mark a 6 if it is *usually true* that you are sly.
Mark a 7 if it is *always or almost always true* that you are sly.

Thus, if you feel it is sometimes but infrequently true that you are "sly," never or almost never true that you are "malicious," always or almost always true that you are "irresponsible," and often true that you are "carefree," then you would rate these characteristics as follows:

Sly	3		Irresponsible	7
Malicious	1		Carefree	5

1   *never or almost never true*
2   *usually not true*
3   *sometimes but infrequently true*
4   *occasionally true*
5   *often true*
6   *usually true*
7   *always or almost always true*

	Rating
Energetic	
Outspoken	
Peaceable	
Self-Confident	
Aggressive	
Quick	
Ambitious	
Calm	
Forceful	
Enterprising	
Headstrong	
Quiet	
Tense	
Enthusiastic	

	Rating
Irritable	
Dominant	
Relaxed	
Assertive	
Argumentative	
Excitable	
Mild	
Loud	
Individualistic	
Easygoing	
Talkative	
Cautious	
Outgoing	
Strong	

Type A's tend to have scores of five to seven in those characteristics typical of the personality type: energetic, outspoken, aggressive, quick, ambitious, forceful, etc., while type B's will have their highest scores in such traits as peaceable, calm, quiet, relaxed, cautious, etc.

STRESS AND HEALTH

Studies have found that illness often occurs at the times of major life events. University of Washington researchers have assigned specific point values to stressful events and correlated them with the likelihood of serious illness or accident. The events may be either tragic or happy; the important thing is the degree of change. As the number of stressful changes a person goes through in a given period of time increases, so does the chance of falling ill. For example, a person who scores between 150 and 300 points has a 50 percent chance of a serious illness within two years; the risk increases to 80 percent if the score is more than 300 points.

The Social Readjustment Rating Scale

Life Event	Value
1. Death of spouse	100
2. Divorce	73
3. Marital separation	65
4. Jail term	63
5. Death of close family member	63
6. Personal injury or illness	53
7. Marriage	50
8. Fired at work	47
9. Marital reconciliation	45
10. Retirement	45
11. Change in health of a family member	44
12. Pregnancy	40
13. Sex difficulties	39
14. Gain of a new family member	39
15. Business readjustment	39
16. Change in financial state	38
17. Death of a close friend	37
18. Change to a different line of work	36
19. Change in number of arguments with spouse	35
20. Mortgage or loan for a major purpose	31
21. Foreclosure of mortgage or loan	30
22. Change in responsibilities at work	29
23. Son or daughter leaving home	29

24. Trouble with in-laws	29
25. Outstanding personal achievement	28
26. Spouse begins or stops work	26
27. Begin or end of school	26
28. Change in living conditions	25
29. Revision of personal habits	24
30. Trouble with boss	23
31. Change in work hours or conditions	20
32. Change in residence	20
33. Change in schools	20
34. Change in recreation	19
35. Change in church activities	19
36. Change in social activities	18
37. Mortgage or loan for a lesser purpose	17
38. Change in sleeping habits	17
39. Change in number of family get-togethers	16
40. Change in eating habits	15
41. Vacation	13
42. Christmas	12
43. Minor violations of the law	11

T. H. Holmes and R. H. Rahe. "The Social Readjustment Scale," *Journal of Psychosomatic Research* Vol. 11, 1967, 213–18 © 1967, Pergamon Press, Inc. Reprinted with permission.

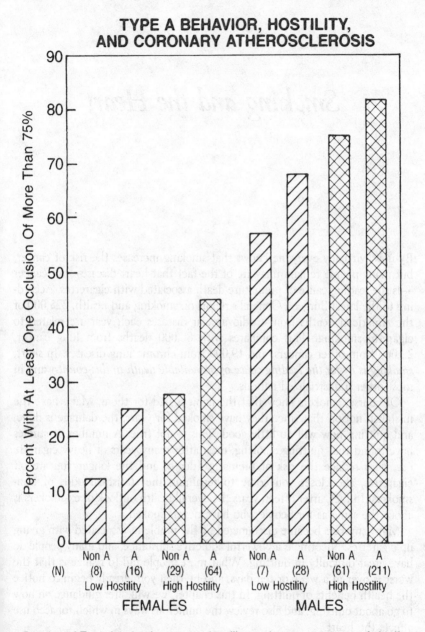

Relation of Type A behavior pattern, hostility, and sex to presence of significant coronary occlusions.

(Adapted from *Psychosomatic Medicine*, Vol. 42, No. 6, page 545, November 1980)

Smoking and the Heart

By now, virtually everyone knows that smoking increases the risk of cancer, but many people remain unaware of the fact that heart disease—not cancer —is the leading cause of premature death associated with cigarettes. According to the latest Surgeon General's report on smoking and health, 225,000 of the American deaths from cardiovascular diseases each year are related to cigarette smoking. This compares with 80,000 deaths from lung cancer, 22,000 from other cancers, and 19,000 from chronic lung diseases. In short, *smoking is by far the leading cause of preventable death in this country* and in most other industrialized nations.

Of course, smokers know that the habit is bad for them. Many have the mistaken notion that since they have smoked for years, the damage is done, and quitting now will do little good. This is not true: A number of studies have found that quitting smoking, even after many years of heavy cigarette use, does reduce the risk of premature death, and the longer you are off cigarettes, the closer you come to regaining the statistical odds of non-smokers. In fact, after fifteen years the overall health outlook of ex-smokers is about the same as for people who have never smoked.

Many smokers became discouraged by the problems associated with giving up cigarettes. Nicotine is a powerful addictive substance, and many people do have great difficulty in quitting. What most people fail to realize is that the worst is over in a week or ten days, and by then you already begin to notice the health benefits of quitting. In this chapter, we will offer guidance on how to go about quitting, and also review the numerous ways in which tobacco use affects the heart.

HOW SMOKING HARMS THE HEART

Tobacco has several major cardiovascular effects that occur almost immediately during smoking. The heart rate increases and blood pressure goes up, meaning that the heart muscle must work even harder to keep the blood circulating. At the same time, however, the amount of oxygen available to the heart is decreased by the very act of smoking. If the coronary arteries already are narrowed by atherosclerotic disease, the heart muscle is even more deprived of vital oxygen. Many experts feel this combination of factors helps explain why smokers are much more vulnerable to heart attacks and to sudden death from cardiac arrhythmias than are nonsmokers.

There are more than four thousand components in tobacco smoke, and probably more that have not been identified. The components include a dozen or so gases, one of the most harmful being carbon monoxide, and particulates, such as tar and nicotine. Not all the mechanisms of how tobacco smoke affects the heart are understood, but recent research has shed considerable light on many of the changes brought on by cigarette smoking.

Nicotine, the main addictive agent in tobacco, has a profound effect on the heart and circulatory system. When nicotine is inhaled, it almost immediately enters the bloodstream. It is a powerful stimulant that, among other things, prompts the adrenal glands to pump out epinephrine (commonly called adrenaline). This is a classic component of the body's "fight-or-flight" response to danger or stress, which causes the heart to beat faster and the blood pressure to rise. Epinephrine is also the most potent known vasopressor, meaning it causes the capillaries and arteries to constrict, or narrow. In addition to raising blood pressure, this reduces the flow of blood to the fingers and toes and other extremities. The reduced blood flow aggravates—or perhaps even causes—a common vascular disorder called Raynaud's disease, which is characterized by faulty circulation to the hands.

Carbon monoxide also has a demonstrated effect on the heart. This odorless gas, which makes up 1 to 5 percent of cigarette smoke, is one of the most poisonous components of tobacco smoke. When inhaled, it sharply reduces the amount of oxygen in the blood. Carbon monoxide has an affinity for hemoglobin—the molecule in the red blood cell that transports oxygen—more than two hundred times greater than that of oxygen. Therefore, when carbon monoxide is present in the lungs, it competes with oxygen in binding, and because of its greater affinity, the carbon monoxide replaces much of the oxygen. When it binds to hemoglobin, a molecule known as carboxyhemoglobin is formed. In the presence of carboxyhemoglobin, oxygen tends to bind even tighter to the hemoglobin. Thus the reduced amount of oxygen in the blood plus the decreased availability of the circulating oxygen to the body cells means that the heart muscle is greatly deprived of much of the oxygen it needs. Studies have found that this combination of events—increased levels of adrenal hormones, increased heart rate and blood pressure, and reduced availability of oxygen—increases the likelihood of angina and serious cardiac arrhythmias.

In addition, carbon monoxide is thought to cause structural changes in the heart and blood vessels. Laboratory studies involving rabbits have found that the gas causes degeneration in the heart muscle itself. Other studies suggest that carboxyhemoglobin makes the blood-vessel walls more permeable to cholesterol and other fats, which may increase their susceptibility to the buildup of fatty deposits. Other researchers have theorized that antigens to components of tobacco smoke may injure the blood-vessel walls, and in this manner promote atherosclerosis. Although further studies are needed to prove these long-term effects, it is increasingly clear that smoking does great harm to the cardiovascular system.

Smoking results in a marked short-term rise in blood pressure, but it is not known whether this leads to sustained hypertension. Hypertensives who smoke, however, have an even greater risk of a heart attack and sudden death than those who do not. In fact, smoking in the presence of any of the other cardiovascular risk factors seems to compound the chances of a heart attack.

IS THERE A SAFE CIGARETTE?

Tobacco manufacturers have markedly lowered the content of both tar and nicotine in cigarettes since the first Surgeon General's report on smoking, in 1964. In addition, filter cigarettes have become much more popular. But are these cigarettes any safer? There is some evidence that they may lower the risk of cancer, but they make little or no difference when it comes to heart disease. In other words, *there is no such thing as a cigarette that is safe for the heart*. In fact, some studies have found that cigarettes with unperforated (unventilated) filters, which reduce the amount of tar, actually increase the amount of carboxyhemoglobin in the blood. There have been several epidemiological studies in which slightly higher cardiovascular death rates have been reported among young men who used this type of filter cigarette, compared to those who used unfiltered brands.

OTHER FORMS OF SMOKING

Most people assume that since pipe and cigar smokers generally do not inhale very much smoke, their risk of smoking-related disease is almost nil. Unfortunately, this is not the case. While pipe and cigar smokers enjoy a somewhat lower risk than cigarette users, they still have a higher incidence of cancer and heart disease than do nonsmokers. For one thing, even though they might not inhale the smoke into their lungs, the amount of smoke in the mouth, larynx, and upper respiratory tract among pipe and cigar smokers is about the same as in cigarette smokers.

A good deal has been written in recent years about the effects of passive or involuntary smoking—the inhaling of other people's tobacco smoke in restaurants, the workplace, cars, airplanes, and other enclosed areas. Two types of smoke—main-stream, which results from the act of smoking, and side-stream, which comes from a smoldering cigarette—are involved in passive smoking. Side-stream smoking has a high concentration of carbon monoxide, and inhaling it can produce carboxyhemoglobin in the passive smoker. Some studies have also suggested that high-risk people—heart patients, infants, people with chronic pulmonary problems—experience an exacerbation of their problems if they are in close contact with smokers or smoke pollution for any length of time. There's also the problem of allergic reactions to tobacco smoke. Tobacco contains a highly allergenic glycoprotein to which about one out of three people are sensitive. In addition to promoting typical allergic reactions—eye irritation, runny nose, difficulty in breathing, or even asthma attacks—sensitivity to this glycoprotein may promote atherosclerosis, according to some studies. The allergic response causes a number of bodily changes, including an increase in the clotting activity (platelet clumping) of the blood. In turn, this is thought to injure the lining of the coronary arteries, making them more susceptible to a buildup of fatty plaque. Although this theory has not yet been proved, some experts feel the evidence is convincing enough to press for even stricter regulation of smoking in public places.

HOW TO GO ABOUT STOPPING

As we said earlier, smokers know that it is bad for their health and most contend they would like to quit. Of course, there are those who understand the risks but feel that smoking affords them enough pleasure to hazard the risks. In these instances, all we can say is stopping has to be an individual decision, and as for those who genuinely want to continue smoking, there's little point in trying to persuade them otherwise. Fortunately, determined smokers are in the minority; most people who smoke really do want to break the habit. An estimated 90 percent of the current smokers have either tried to stop or would like to quit if there were an easy way of doing so. This discussion, then, is directed to the many people who want to quit but either don't know how to go about it or become overly discouraged by the difficulties they encounter.

Since the first Surgeon General's report on smoking was released, more than 30 million Americans have quit smoking. Unfortunately, many of these have been replaced by new smokers, so the total numbers are not markedly different: about 50 million Americans smoke. There have been changes in the types of people who smoke. Large numbers of men, particularly those who are in the middle to upper income groups, have quit smoking. Of particular note is the large number of doctors who have stopped smoking. But, in the past decade or so, there has been a marked increase in smoking among women and adolescents. As a result of these shifts, some disturbing trends regarding women's health statistics are beginning to emerge. There is a marked increase, for example, in lung cancer among women—a malignancy that was exceedingly rare in this group only a few years ago. Now it is estimated that, within the next three or four years, lung cancer will surpass breast cancer and become the leading cause of cancer death in women—a situation that has prevailed for several decades for men. There is also an increase in heart attacks among women; most experts agree that this is undoubtedly due to a combination of factors, but the rise in the number of women smoking is certainly high on the list of possible explanations. Unfortunately, much of the tobacco advertising message is now directed to women, while very little of the emphasis on quitting is directed to them.

Of people who quit smoking, the large majority—about 95 percent—manage to do it on their own. Since nicotine is a powerful addictive substance, no one argues that quitting is not difficult. The longer and more heavily you smoke, the harder it is to quit. People who start smoking when they are very young often find quitting more difficult than those who took up the habit later in life. Also, women seem to find it more difficult to quit than men. Light smokers (less than half a pack a day) or people who must stop smoking because of their health seem to have the least difficulty quitting.

The biggest difficulties encountered when stopping are an uncomfortable craving for cigarettes, increased irritability, jittery nerves, anxiety, and inability to concentrate. Although these withdrawal symptoms are common, they are by no means universal; up to 40 to 50 percent of smokers are pleasantly surprised to find they experience no or very minor symptoms. And those who do have withdrawal problems should take heart in the fact that it takes the body only three to seven days to rid itself of most of the nicotine, meaning that the worst is usually over in ten days. A few people will continue to crave cigarettes for a longer period, and some others may experience nervousness and other symptoms but diminishing in intensity. These adverse feelings are offset by the very real health benefits that become noticeable within a few days of stopping. For example, the characteristic smoker's cough begins to diminish within a few days; breathing becomes easier, and the senses of taste and smell recover. Many former smokers express amazement that once again they are able to discern subtle food flavors and smell flowers and food. In their advice to DUPAC patients, Dr. Robert H. Shipley, who developed the program for the Duke Quit Smoking Clinic, and Dr. Carole Orleans, sum up the benefits of quitting by saying, "The quality of your life will rapidly improve if you invest the work and time necessary to be an ex-smoker. . . . You'll breath easier, have more energy on less sleep, have a younger complexion, rid yourself of cigarette odors, be able to taste and smell better, sleep better, and digest your food better with less stomach upset. You'll have a lower heart rate and be able to work harder with less sweat. Perhaps more important, when you quit smoking you will feel justifiably proud of freeing yourself of an enslaving addiction, and for presenting a good example to your children. As part of the bargain, you will also drastically reduce your risk of suffering dread diseases, such as heart attacks, lung cancer, bronchitis and emphysema. Best of all, you'll feel better as a nonsmoker."

Enough said about the benefits of quitting; the big question is how best to go about achieving it. Unfortunately, no one way works best for all people. The highest success rate comes from quitting "cold turkey." Those who find this impossible often succeed with group support and the financial commitment involved in attending a commercial stop-smoking clinic. There are also a number of free or low-cost smoking-cessation programs sponsored by organizations such as the American Heart Association, the American Cancer Society, the Seventh-Day Adventist Church, and others. Hypnosis works for some people, and others benefit from behavior-modification or smoke-aversion sessions. No matter what method you select, planning is an important element in your ultimate success. As Drs. Orleans and Shipley emphasize, "Quitting is not just a matter of having willpower; it is also a matter of using systematic methods to head off smoking urges or to ride them out when they occur." Specific steps they recommend for DUPAC patients include:

Expect to succeed. Talk to friends who are ex-smokers; they can tell you what to expect and give you helpful advice on how to get through any rough times. Anticipate the benefits from quitting; you may even want to make a list of them and post it in a prominent place for added motivation.

Analyze your smoking habit. For at least two days, keep a smoking diary. Note each time you light a cigarette and the circumstances, including how you feel both before and after smoking. You should soon begin to notice a definite pattern of time, place, emotional framework, and associated activities. Note, too, the situations in which you rarely smoke.

Avoid high-risk smoking situations, at least in the beginning. For example, if you invariably smoke when you play cards or during a coffee break, temporarily find other diversions. Go to the movies, take a walk, or engage in other activities that are not associated with smoking. Some situations are more difficult to avoid. For instance, many people end each meal with a cup of coffee and a cigarette. You may temporarily have to plan a new meal-end ritual.

Set a target date for quitting. If you plan to quit cold turkey, give yourself three or four weeks of planning time. Pick a date that does not coincide with a stressful period: tax time, a change in job, any anticipated trying time. Instead, plan less stressful activities for the first week or so.

Reduce nicotine dependency. Cravings for cigarettes are closely related to the level of nicotine in your body. Drs. Orleans and Shipley stress that, ultimately, the best way to stop is cold turkey, because withdrawal symptoms are less severe and drawn out when all smoking is stopped. Also, most people cannot get below ten or twelve cigarettes a day by gradually cutting back. However, nicotine dependency can be minimized before quitting by one of two strategies. "First, you can gradually cut down to 10 to 12 cigarettes a day, and practice coping with resisted smoking urges," Drs. Orleans and Shipley advise. "But then quit abruptly without trying to further gradually reduce your smoking."

The second nicotine-fading strategy involves switching to brands with increasingly less nicotine without cutting back on the number of cigarettes smoked. Try cutting your nicotine intake by 30 percent of your usual level each week until you reach 10 percent of that level. Then quit abruptly. Obviously, this approach applies only if you are not already smoking the lowest-nicotine brands.

Pay attention to your diet. During the quitting phase, eat a balanced high-protein diet and avoid sugary or starch snacks, which raise blood-sugar levels but then cause them to drop, creating the so-called "sugar blues," which are often associated with cigarette craving. Cut down on coffee and other stimulants. If you are worried about gaining weight—many people who quit gain five to ten pounds in the first few weeks due to changes in metabolism and, more important, changed food habits—make sure that you have plenty of low-calorie snacks handy.

Increase your exercise. Exercise not only helps calm jittery nerves and re-

lieve tension, it also controls your appetite and thereby helps prevent unwanted weight gain. It also makes you feel better, both physically and psycho-
logically—important factors in avoiding the temptation to smoke.

Smoke-proof your home and work area. Remove all ashtrays and get rid of
all cigarettes, including reserve packs you may have stashed away. Post
"Thank you for not smoking" signs in your office, and if a guest or compan-
ion asks, "Do you mind if I smoke?" don't be afraid to say, "Yes." Eventually
you may be able to resist such temptations, but why subject yourself to them
when you are trying to give up the habit?

Experiment with smoking substitutes. For many people, smoking is a nervous habit. Common substitutes include doodling, fingering worry beads,
chewing gum, sucking on a low-calorie candy, chewing a toothpick or Stim-
U-Dent, munching on carrot sticks or celery, and working crossword puzzles.
"Choose substitutes that make sense for you," Drs. Orleans and Shipley
advise. "Don't expect the replacement to be as enjoyable as smoking in the
beginning, but over time, the activities can become just as relaxing and
enjoyable. After all, smoking in the beginning is not all that enjoyable
either."

Enlist the aid of friends and family. Many people try to "go it alone,"
perhaps because they don't want to risk public failure. "Smoking is a tough
habit to break," Drs. Orleans and Shipley remind DUPAC participants. "We
recommend asking close friends and family to offer daily support or encouragement in ways you feel will be helpful." At the very least, they add, you
should ask people not to offer you cigarettes, to praise and encourage your
successes, and to ignore any slips.

Expect an occasional backsliding. It takes a very strong person to resist all
temptations, and to never slip up, especially when it comes to breaking a
firmly established smoking habit. The vast majority of ex-smokers experience
an occasional reversal. But those who eventually succeed look upon it as a
temporary slip and promptly resume their effort to quit. Concentrate on your
successes, rather than the failures: "I've gone two entire days without smoking" is a much more positive approach than "I've broken down four times in
the last week and will probably never be able to fully shake the habit." Even a
resumption in smoking should not be viewed as a total failure; studies have
found that each successive attempt to quit is likely to be more successful than
previous attempts. At least 70 percent of those who have successfully quit
admit to at least one earlier, unsuccessful attempt, and some people quit a
dozen or more times before they shake the habit once and for all.

STOP-SMOKING CLINICS

About 30 percent of those smokers who say they want to quit feel they could benefit from a formal stop-smoking program, according to a report by the American Cancer Society. Yet only a small percentage actually sign up for such a program. A reason commonly cited for this in the past was the lack of availability of stop-smoking programs. This has changed in recent years, however, as a growing number of organizations, ranging from the American Cancer Society and the American Heart Association to community hospitals, employers, and commercial groups such as SmokEnders, have expanded their activities throughout the country. Almost everyone who now wants to join a stop-smoking program can find one within his or her geographic area. For specific information and guidance, ask your doctor about stop-smoking programs or contact your local chapter of the American Cancer Society or the American Heart Association. These two voluntary organizations keep directories of stop-smoking programs and can tell you what is involved and also give particulars on enrolling.

The success rate—the number of people who actually manage to stop smoking and have not resumed the habit six months to a year later—is lower than that of people who quit on their own. A program with a 30 to 50 percent success rate is considered very good indeed.

The foci of stop-smoking clinics vary considerably. Those run by voluntary health organizations, such as the American Cancer Society, tend to emphasize health education and group support. A typical ACS program consists of a four-week course, with two 1 1/2 hour sessions a week. The course is divided into three phases: analysis of the smoking habit, practicing quitting in controlled situations, and maintaining cigarette abstinence. Participants learn how to cope with withdrawal symptoms and to avoid situations that are likely to lead to smoking. A buddy support system also is incorporated, and nonsmoking is rewarded.

Another major nonsmoking effort is conducted by the Seventh-Day Adventist Church, which offers stop-smoking clinics for the general public. Theirs is a five-day plan, with two-hour sessions on five consecutive days. A buddy support system is used, and much of the focus is on health education and learning to deal with tobacco withdrawal. Coping techniques include learning deep breathing exercises to control tension, increasing water intake, and reducing coffee consumption.

Stop-smoking clinics have become an important element in many workplace health programs. These have several advantages: they are convenient to attend, they offer peer support from among colleagues, and the endorsement of the employer is an added incentive. Many are conducted by outside commercial clinics or medical facilities, and are offered free or at a moderate fee to employees. If your company has not yet offered such a program and there are enough employees interested in enrolling, talk to your personnel or medical department. Numerous studies have demonstrated that smokers have many more sick days each year. A survey by the U.S. Public Health Service estimated that smokers have an extra 81 million sick days per year and spend 145 million extra days in bed over those of nonsmokers. The economic toll is tremendous; the American Medical Association estimates that up to 25 percent of the nation's total medical bill, now approaching $300 billion, is directly related to smoking. This may be as high as $75 billion a year, or more than $300 for each man, woman, and child in the United States. Since many of these costs fall directly on employers, either through increased medical and insurance costs or lost workdays and lowered productivity, most companies are very eager to have their employees stop smoking, and will support on-site programs.

Other formal stop-smoking programs are available from hospitals, health-maintenance organizations, and other medical groups. At Duke, the Quit Smoking Clinic is part of the Behavior Change and Self-Control Program. The clinic is staffed by clinical psychologists and other trained specialists, all of whom recognize the difficulty in breaking the smoking habit. Treatment involves five sessions spread over eight days. Participants are instructed not to smoke during the treatment program except during the actual session. At that time, they will be instructed in smoking in such a way that the desire to smoke will be reduced. Other aspects of the treatment include the use of subliminal support messages that increase self-control, and relaxation training aimed at increasing resistance to the urge to smoke. Other aspects of the treatment are tailored to the personality and smoking pattern of the individual.

In the past decade, a number of commercial stop-smoking groups also have emerged. SmokEnders is one of the oldest and largest of these. It emphasizes a gradual reduction technique and rewards accomplishments. The course involves nine weekly sessions—participants may request additional sessions if needed. By the fifth week, participants are instructed to stop smoking completely. Fees range from three hundred dollars up and are considered an added motivation to stop: "If you want to stop badly enough to pay for it, you're more likely to succeed," says Jacquelyn Rogers, cofounder of SmokEnders and author of a highly recommended book, *You Can Stop.* SmokEnders, perhaps because its participants are highly motivated, enjoys a high success rate: 35 to 55 percent of its graduates are still off cigarettes at the end of one year.

Smoke Watchers, a group patterned somewhat on Weight Watchers, assigns weekly smoke-reduction goals until the member stops completely. Enrollment involves paying a membership fee and then an additional fee for each weekly session.

Some commercial clinics employ various behavior-modification techniques. The Schick Centers for the Control of Smoking, for example, use smoke-aversion training, which requires participants to oversmoke by puffing very rapidly until the smoking experience becomes very unpleasant. Mild electric shocks are also used to destroy the pleasant aspects of smoking. The initial treatments, which emphasize the oversmoking, are given on five consecutive days, followed by sixteen twice-weekly sessions for further educational and general support. The fee is somewhat high: five hundred dollars for the course. However, if the participant has not stopped smoking by the fifth session, a refund is offered.

Although smoke-aversion training works for some people, *it is not generally recommended for people who have heart or lung disorders.* Therefore, you should check with your doctor before enrolling in any course that involves oversmoking.

Hypnosis is another technique employed by some commercial programs. Since this should be done under the supervision of a qualified medical hypnotist, it is not as widely available as programs that can be conducted by trained lay leaders. If you think hypnosis may work for you, ask your doctor to recommend a reliable practitioner who offers this approach.

THE ROLE OF YOUR DOCTOR

Studies have found that even a brief conversation with your doctor can markedly increase your chances of stopping smoking. A two-minute discussion during which the doctor encourages a patient to give up smoking and suggests methods that might be most effective for that particular individual results in an average 3 percent cessation rate. The rate nearly doubles if the doctor spends four minutes discussing the health benefits of stopping and also gives the patient literature on how to go about it. Compounded over a number of years, such physician counseling could have a major impact on reducing the total number of smokers.

SMOKING PREVENTION PROGRAMS

Of course, the most effective method of all is to never take up the habit in the first place. Studies have found that most people start smoking at an early age—twelve to fourteen have been identified as the most vulnerable years. Therefore, smoking prevention programs in the schools should be an important part of the national strategy in reducing the number of tobacco users. Yet a surprising number of schools fail to offer smoking prevention programs, claiming that the funds for such "frills" are not available. This is one area in which parents should investigate what is offered at their children's schools, and if no smoking prevention programs are included in the curriculum, they should request that they be added. One such program, the University of Minnesota Smoking Prevention Program, has been developed and carefully tested in the Minneapolis-area schools for more than five years. It enlists student leaders to direct the sessions and focuses on areas that are of most concern to youngsters—things like bad breath from smoking, lessened endurance for sports, offensiveness to others—rather than the long-term health consequences of smoking. More information may be obtained by contacting the University of Minnesota School of Public Health, Stadium Station, University of Minnesota School of Medicine, Minneapolis, Minn. 55455.

ONCE YOU HAVE QUIT

As noted earlier, many people quit smoking but then take up the habit again in a few weeks or months. Thus, it's not enough to simply quit; it's also important to remain a nonsmoker.

Most people relapse in the first three months of quitting. According to Drs. Orleans and Shipley, it is not just the constant temptation that leads to the backsliding; instead, it is the inability to cope with anger, frustration, or tension that generally leads to a resumption of smoking. Some people lack the confidence to stay off cigarettes, or think they can have just one or two and it won't matter. Situations that involve a good deal of tension—"Just one cigarette will help me get through the presentation" or "I'll be able to concentrate on the test if I have just one cigarette first"—are common examples.

To overcome in such situations, you should be prepared with specific coping techniques. Practice the relaxation exercises outlined on pages 155–58, or "take a breather" when you are under tension. This involves assuming a comfortable position and then placing one hand on your chest and the other on your abdomen. Take a deep breath through your nose, hold it for a few seconds, and then slowly let it out through your mouth with a slight blowing motion. Say the word "relax" to yourself, and repeat twenty to thirty times. Do this two or three times a day, or when faced with situations in which you are sorely tempted to light a cigarette. You'll be surprised at how it helps dissolve tension and remove the longing for a cigarette.

THE QUESTION OF WEIGHT GAIN

Many people fear they will gain unwanted weight once they stop smoking, and many people do put on five to ten pounds in the first few weeks after quitting. Some people who substitute snacking on high-calorie foods for smoking may gain considerably more. If weight gain is a problem, it should not be construed as an excuse to resume smoking. Instead, concentrate on effective weight-control techniques. Have plenty of low-calorie snacks on hand. An apple can be just as satisfying as a candy bar, and it has a lot fewer calories and provides important nutrients. Food will taste better after you stop smoking, and your appetite will improve. Learn to modify your portions.

Increasing your exercise will also help curb your appetite, control weight gain, and relieve the tension created by not smoking. Above all, the fear of gaining weight should not keep you from quitting smoking. If you find you are gaining weight, apply the weight-control advice outlined in the chapter "Diet and the Heart." And as DUPAC's Paul Koisch likes to point out, it takes fifty excess pounds of weight to match the negative health effects of smoking!

SUMMING UP

Cigarette smoking is a major risk factor in heart attacks and other forms of heart disease. According to the latest Surgeon General's report on smoking and health, an estimated 225,000 cardiac deaths a year are directly related to smoking, and it is the leading cause of preventable premature death in this country. One of the most important things a smoker—particularly one with heart disease—can do is to stop. Although many people experience unpleasant withdrawal symptoms during the first few days after stopping, these tend to be short-lived. And up to 40 to 50 percent of former smokers report that they managed to quit with little or no withdrawal symptoms. In this chapter we have reviewed the important health benefits to be deprived from quitting and have also outlined steps and resources you might employ in breaking your own cigarette habit.

For more material and information on how to go about quitting, you can obtain a *Helping Smokers Quit Kit* from the National Cancer Institute. To obtain a kit, write the Office of Cancer Communications, National Cancer Institute, Bethesda, Md. 20205. Local chapters of the American Lung Association offer two manuals, *Freedom from Smoking in 20 Days* and *A Lifetime of Freedom from Smoking.* Local chapters are listed in the telephone white pages, or you may write to the national office: American Lung Association, 1740 Broadway, New York, N.Y. 10019.

Most experts agree that the smoking habit is one that is difficult to break. But the health benefits begin almost immediately, and the worst is generally over within two weeks. If you truly want to quit smoking, there's no reason why you can't become one of the many millions who have stopped. And if you do backslide, resist the temptation to call the whole effort a failure and take up smoking as before. Instead, concentrate on the successes and, if need be, start over again. Remember, millions of people who can now call themselves ex-smokers report that they stopped two, three, or more times before finally quitting completely.

Returning to Work: The Need for Vocational Rehabilitation

Brad C. loved his job as a Durham fireman. Ever since he was a boy, he had wanted to be a fireman, and as soon as he completed his education, he took the test for fire-fighting trainees. "I still look back on the day I joined the fire company as one of the happiest in my life," he says. But, at age thirty-three, his fire-fighting career was over, ended by two severe heart attacks.

Brad is by no means unique; more than a half million Americans under the age of sixty-five are receiving disability benefits because of cardiovascular disease. In fact, cardiovascular diseases are by far the leading cause of premature retirement and disability in this country, costing the national economy an estimated $12.4 billion a year. Yet a number of studies have found that many, if not most, of those declared too disabled to work or are forced to take an early retirement could, with proper cardiac and vocational rehabilitation, be employed. In the case of Brad, he was able to be reassigned to a less physically demanding desk job with the Durham police department. It may not be his first choice, but it enables him to continue to support his family and is not so far removed from his old job as to require total retraining or additional education.

Of course, not everyone who has a heart attack requires extensive rehabilitation. There are many patients who return to work in two or three months without any problems; a good deal depends on the nature of the work and the individual's physical condition. If the job involves a good deal of stress or physical exertion, some adjustments or changes may be required. Other considerations include the safety of others, as is the case with airline pilots, who usually are barred from flying following a heart attack. But just because a former pilot may no longer be able to fly a plane, this does not mean that his talent and experience cannot be used in a ground-based job.

Successful vocational rehabilitation often requires a concerted effort of the patient, the physician and other medical therapists, the employer, and in some instances, trained vocational counselors. In many cases, there is a great temptation to take the easy way out and claim disability. After a heart attack, most patients want to return to work. But as the seriousness of the disease becomes more clear, this eagerness to resume working begins to erode. Perhaps the job involved more drudgery than satisfaction, or maybe it is blamed for causing the heart attack. The disability benefits may be on a par with former earnings, removing any financial incentive to return to work. Doubts and confusion are often reinforced by physicians who will usually go along with the patient's wishes and recommend an early retirement or permanent disability, rather than elect referral for rehabilitation. The net result is that large numbers of people who are still capable of leading productive lives are instead classified as cardiac cripples and relegated to a dependent, rather than an independent, role. This, of course, does not apply to those whose disease is so severe that they are unable to work; obviously, they should not be pressured into resuming a job that may be injurious to them or to others. It should be noted, however, that even people severely limited by their disease can benefit from cardiac rehabilitation, even if it is clear they will not return to their jobs.

North Carolina has one of the nation's most progressive rehabilitation programs. The State Department of Human Resources has licensed twelve cardiac rehabilitation programs—including DUPAC—making them eligible for insurance benefits. At first, the insurance industry was skeptical that exercise conditioning could be an effective means of returning heart patients to their jobs, but the success of DUPAC and similar programs has disproved this.

Putting the Lessons
of DUPAC to Work for You

In the preceeding chapters, we have described the various components of
DUPAC, along with their medical and scientific rationale. The important
question, of course, is, How do you go about putting these principles into
practice in your own life? As emphasized earlier, if you have heart disease,
you should see your doctor first. If you are a healthy but sedentary person,
you also should undergo a medical checkup before embarking on exercise
conditioning. This is particularly important if you have any symptoms of
heart disease or strong risk factors; namely, if you have high blood pressure or
high cholesterol, are overweight, smoke, or have a family history of early
heart attacks. If you are a healthy person who already exercises but would like
to follow the DUPAC regimen, it is probably safe. In any instance, use
common sense and heed any warnings from your body.

While it is quite possible to follow the DUPAC—or any other exercise-
conditioning/cardiovascular-rehabilitation program—on your own, most people who have been through the DUPAC experience agree that it has given
them a unique insight into both their disease and the most effective means of
overcoming it. Gerald S., the New York professor who spent a month at
DUPAC following a heart attack and bypass surgery, explains it this way:
"There is something about the esprit de corps and companionship with both
your fellow patients and the medical staff that gives you the motivation to
extend your limits. You need to know how much you can do, and then with
the help and support of those around you, find the courage to do it. We often
forget that after a heart attack, you are very afraid of testing yourself. And if
you don't feel good in addition to being afraid, there's an even greater temptation to simply take your drugs and resign yourself to being a semi-invalid."

This does not mean that the only alternative is to pack your bags and head
for the Duke Medical Center (although people do come from throughout the
United States to participate in DUPAC). Given the proper understanding

and guidance from your own doctor, you can rehabilitate yourself. You don't need a special facility or equipment to undertake a graduated walking/jogging program. You can assess your diet and determine what should be changed to bring it in line with the prudent one recommended by DUPAC, the American Heart Association, and most doctors. You can identify points of stress and learn more effective coping techniques and ways of relaxing. You can stop smoking, even if you have been a heavy tobacco user for many years. None of this is terribly difficult or mysterious; motivation and common sense are the most important ingredients.

There are also a large number of effective cardiovascular rehabilitation programs throughout the country. Many are based in medical centers or hospitals; some are even modeled on DUPAC or incorporate very similar programs. Others may be run by a local YMCA, individual physicians, or even commercial health-and-fitness centers. In assessing whether one of these rehabilitation programs might be appropriate for you, use the following checklist:

1. Does it require a physician referral? This would indicate that a recognized medical endorsement is important. If you have heart disease, it's important that people overseeing your rehabilitation efforts be familiar with your medical history. If you have any doubts, ask your own doctor.

2. Is a complete medical workup, including an exercise tolerance test, included in the preliminary phase? This should be a requirement for anyone with established heart disease or a sedentary person with a suspicion of hidden disease.

3. Are you given a rehabilitation program individualized to meet your particular needs? While you may be working out with everyone else, it is still important that you know your own training heart rate and your own individualized exercise prescription.

4. Are trained medical personnel and emergency equipment at all exercise sessions? They may never be called upon, but they still should be on hand just in case.

5. Are you comfortable with the supervisors, your fellow participants, the setting? Group support is a very important factor in a rehabilitative effort, particularly one that involves such a serious health problem as heart disease.

6. Is the program one that can be adapted to your schedule and life? It's one thing to enroll in a rehabilitation program and "get back on your feet," and quite another to follow it for the rest of your life. Heart disease is a lifelong disease, and living with it has to be a lifelong effort.

7. Is there a total approach? Many rehabilitation programs focus on only one or two aspects: exercise conditioning, psychological counseling, relaxation

techniques, diet, etc. The most successful are likely to be those that promote a prudent total approach that encompasses all of these.

8. Does it make unrealistic promises? Some programs promise that you will be able to throw away your drugs, get in shape without expending any physical effort, be cured of your disease. Such promises should be viewed with considerable skepticism.

Other factors, such as insurance reimbursement, cost, and location also should be considered. Many companies now support cardiac rehabilitation for their employees. If yours does not, you might want to talk to your personnel or medical director about instituting a health-promotion program that incorporates exercise conditioning, nutrition counseling, stop-smoking clinics, behavior-modification and relaxation training, and other elements of cardiac conditioning.

Of course, you don't have to wait for a heart attack or other symptoms of heart disease to embark on a conditioning program. Although DUPAC was originally developed for heart patients, almost everyone can benefit from its lessons and example. Even the most sedentary people can be induced to change their ways. The most compulsive Type A personalities can enjoy a less frantic but fully productive life-style. And even those with markedly impaired heart function can regain control over their lives and benefit from a well-supervised and individually tailored conditioning program.

Glossary

Aneurysm

A weakening of a blood vessel, usually an artery, due to disease, traumatic injury, or congenital abnormality, leading to a ballooning and sometimes rupture of the vessel wall.

Angina pectoris

Chest pain caused by a temporary lack of oxygen to the heart. The condition is usually caused by coronary atherosclerosis, or chronic narrowing of the arteries to the heart. It can also be caused by low oxygen levels in the blood, restricted blood flow to the heart, coronary spasm, or overexertion.

Angiocardiogram

A chest X ray taken after the injection of a dye into the bloodstream for viewing the inside dimensions of the heart and its arteries.

Antiarrhythmic Drugs

Drugs used to restore proper heart rate and rhythm in patients suffering from arrhythmias.

Anticoagulant

A drug that delays blood clotting but does not dissolve already existing blood clots.

Antihypertensive Drugs

Drugs used to control hypertension, or high blood pressure, by slowing the heartbeat, eliminating excess fluids, or dilating the arteries.

Aorta

The main artery (leading away from the heart), which receives blood from the left ventricle of the heart. It arches over the heart and branches with the aorta carrying blood down through the chest and abdomen, while the carotid artery carries blood upward to the brain.

Aortic stenosis

A narrowing of the valve, or opening, between the left ventricle of the heart and the aorta.

Aortic valve
The valve between the aorta and the left ventricle of the heart, which allows blood to flow from the heart into the aorta but not back into the heart.

Arrhythmia
A variation from the normal heart-rate rhythm.

Arterial blood
Blood that is oxygenated in the lungs and then flows to the left side of the heart through the pulmonary veins. From there, the oxygenated blood is pumped through the left side of the heart into the arteries and then throughout the bloodstream.

Arterioles
The smallest of the arterial vessels (diameter 1/125 inch). Their function is to pass blood from the arteries to the capillaries.

Arteriosclerosis
A thickening and loss of elasticity of the artery walls, which cuts down on blood flow and strains the heart. The condition is attributed to an accumulation of fibrous tissue, cholesterol, or other material.

Atheroma
A deposit of fatty substances in the inner lining of the artery wall, sometimes called plaque.

Atherosclerosis
A thickening of the artery wall due to deposits of fatty substances, causing a narrowing of the artery. This is one type of arteriosclerosis.

Atrium
One of the two upper chambers of the heart, formerly known as the auricles. The right atrium receives unoxygenated blood from the body, and the left atrium receives oxygenated blood from the lungs ready for circulation.

Autonomic nervous system
The involuntary nervous system, consisting of the sympathetic and the parasympathetic nerves, which regulate body tissue and function. The sympathetic nerves tend to increase heart rate, while the parasympathetic nerves tend to slow heart rate and lower blood pressure, when stimulated.

Bacterial endocarditis
A bacterial infection of the inner layer of the heart causing inflammation of the lining of the heart valves.

Biofeedback
A technique for helping control the involuntary systems within the body through visualization of body functions. The use of lights and projected images depicting blood pressure, heart rate, gastrointestinal activity, and other normally involuntary

functions have been highly successful in helping the patient control his biological systems.

BLOOD PRESSURE
The force exerted by circulating blood against the artery walls. Blood-pressure measurements reflect the systolic pressure, based on contractions, over the diastolic pressure, reflecting the relaxation of the heart. A typical blood-pressure reading (in the normal range) might be 120/80.

CALORIE
A unit of energy representing the amount of heat required to raise the temperature of one kilogram of water one degree Celsius. Calories are used as a measurement of how much energy is present in foods.

CAPILLARIES
The smallest of all the blood vessels, capillaries pass oxygen and nutrients to all body tissues while removing carbon dioxide and waste products.

CARDIAC OUTPUT
The amount of blood pumped by the heart per minute.

CARDIAC RESERVE
The difference between the resting cardiac output and the output during maximum physical exertion. The difference can be as much as five times, rising from five quarts per minute to twenty-five quarts per minute or more.

CARDIOMYOPATHY
Disease involving the myocardium, or heart muscle, caused by either known or unknown toxic or infectious agents.

CARDIOPULMONARY RESUSCITATION (CPR)
An emergency treatment that can be performed by one or two people to maintain a patient's circulation until medical help arrives. Also called basic life support, CPR can artificially maintain breathing and circulation through external cardiac compression and artificial respiration in the event of cardiac arrest, drowning, or other emergency.

CAROTID ARTERIES
The principal arteries supplying blood to the head and neck, one on each side of the neck. Each has two branches, internal and external. The external carotid artery is close to the surface and may be felt for taking one's own heart rate.

CATHETER
A thin, flexible tube that can be inserted deep into body organs for use in diagnosis, treatment, or drainage. A cardiac catheter is inserted into the heart, its progress watched on a fluoroscope, for use in diagnosis or treatment.

CATHETERIZATION
The insertion of a catheter.

Collateral circulation
A detouring of the blood through smaller vessels when a main blood vessel has been blocked off.

Congestive heart failure
Congestion in the body tissues caused by a failure of the heart to pump its normal amount of blood, leading to accumulation of fluid in the abdomen, legs, and/or lungs. This condition can develop over a period of years, although attacks can be short and severe. It is generally treated with drugs or, if necessary, surgically.

Coronary arteries
The arteries that conduct blood to the heart muscle, rising from the base of the aorta and coming down over the top of the heart like a crown, or corona.

Coronary-artery bypass surgery
A surgical operation in which veins (or sometimes arteries) are taken from other parts of the body (usually the leg) and grafted onto the heart to construct detours through which oxygenated blood can travel to the heart muscle. It is performed on patients whose coronary arteries are severely narrowed (reducing blood flow to the heart and usually causing chest pain and increased risk of heart attack). It is sometimes performed following a heart attack to decrease the chances of repeated heart failure.

Coronary atherosclerosis
Known as coronary heart disease, this is a narrowing of the coronary arteries caused by thickening of the inner layer of the arterial walls (which reduces the blood supply to the heart muscle).

Coronary heart disease
A narrowing of the coronary arteries leading to a decreased blood supply to the heart. Also known as coronary artery disease and ischemic heart disease.

Coronary insufficiency
Insufficient delivery of oxygen to the heart, often causing chest pain (angina pectoris) or heart attack.

Coronary occlusion
An obstruction in one of the coronary arteries which hinders the blood flow to the heart muscle, causing a portion of the heart muscle to be destroyed because of lack of oxygen (heart attack).

Coronary thrombosis
A clot in an artery blocking blood flow to the heart muscle.

Cyanosis
Blueness of the skin caused by insufficient oxygenation of the blood.

Defibrillation
A treatment, usually by electric shock, to stop atrial or ventricular arrythmias, or fibrillation.

DIASTOLE
The period of relaxation in each heartbeat.

DILATION
A widening of the heart or blood vessels beyond the norm.

DIURETIC
A drug used to remove excess body fluids by promoting salt excretion.

DYSPNEA
Shortness of breath.

ELECTROCARDIOGRAM
Commonly known as EKG, or ECG, this is a test which graphically records the electric currents generated by the heart. Results of the test reveal heart rate and certain abnormalities, such as undersupply of blood or enlargement of heart chambers.

EPINEPHRINE
Adrenaline produced and secreted by the adrenal glands, situated just above the kidneys. This hormone constricts the small blood vessels, increases heart rate, and raises blood pressure.

ESSENTIAL HYPERTENSION
High blood pressure of an unknown cause.

EXERCISE ELECTROCARDIOGRAM
Also called a stress test, this is administered while the patient is exercising, usually on a treadmill or an exercise bicycle, to record the electric currents generated by the heart in order to monitor heart function.

FIBRILLATION
Uncoordinated contraction of the heart muscle—a type of cardiac arrhythmia.

HEART BLOCK
A blockage or slowing of the electrical impulse within the heart's conduction system, causing uncoordinated rhythms of the upper and the lower heart chambers. This can be corrected with an artificial pacemaker.

HEART FAILURE
A condition in which the heart is unable to pump enough blood to maintain normal blood circulation. It may be due to circulatory disorder, high blood pressure, rheumatic heart disease, birth defect, or heart attack.

HEMOGLOBIN
The oxygen-carrying, red pigment of the red blood cells. Hemoglobin absorbs oxygen in the lungs, becoming bright red and is then called oxyhemoglobin. After some of the oxygen has been distributed to body tissues, the hemoglobin turns dark burgundy and is called reduced hemoglobin.

HYPERCHOLESTEROLEMIA
An excess of cholesterol, or fatty substances, in the blood.

HYPERLIPOPROTEINEMIA
An excess of lipoproteins—complexes of fatty substances called lipids and certain proteins—in the blood.

HYPERTENSION
High blood pressure.

HYPOTENSION
Low blood pressure.

HYPOXIA
Lack of oxygen in the organs and tissues of the body.

INFARCT
The area of tissue that is permanently damaged, or dies, as a result of lack of blood and oxygen supply.

ISCHEMIA
Temporary oxygen deficiency in a localized part of the body, caused by an obstruction in the blood vessel.

ISCHEMIC HEART DISEASE
Heart ailments caused by narrowing of the coronary arteries and a resultant decrease in blood supply to the heart. Also called coronary artery disease or coronary heart disease.

LIPOPROTEIN
A complex of lipid and protein molecules bound together. Lipids are fatty substances that are not water soluble.

MURMUR
An extra heart sound heard between the normal heartbeats. This is a common condition which is generally harmless.

MYOCARDIAL INFARCTION
Permanent damage, or death, of an area of the myocardium, or heart muscle, resulting from lack of blood and oxygen supply.

MYOCARDIUM
The muscular wall of the heart.

NOREPINEPHRINE
Also called noradrenaline, this organic compound raises blood pressure by constricting the small blood vessels.

PACEMAKER
The origin of electrical impulses that initiate contractions of the heart. The pacemaker is an organic mass of specialized cells situated in the right atrium of the heart. If the pacemaker becomes damaged, it can be replaced by an artificial pacemaker (internal or external), which electrically substitutes for the natural pacemaker in controlling the rhythm of heartbeats.

PALPITATION
An abnormal heart rate, indicated by a sensation of fluttering around the heart area.

PLATELETS
Small, disk-shaped bodies found in the blood that are instrumental in the formation of blood clots.

REGURGITATION
Backward flow through a defective valve. In cardiology, refers to the backward flow of blood.

REVASCULARIZATION
A surgical operation to restore normal blood flow to body tissues by removing the thickened inner lining of narrowed arteries or by rerouting blood through other vessels already in place or grafted into place from other parts of the body. Coronary bypass surgery is a type of revascularization.

SCLEROSIS
Hardening or thickening, as in arteriosclerosis, or hardening of the arteries.

SINUS RHYTHM
Normal heart rhythm initiated in the sinoatrial node, or pacemaker.

SPHYGMOMANOMETER
An instrument used for measuring blood pressure in the arteries.

STENOSIS
A narrowing of an opening such as a valve.

SYNCOPE
The act of fainting, often caused by insufficient blood and oxygen to the brain.

SYSTOLE
The period of contraction of the heart in each heartbeat.

TACHYCARDIA
Abnormally fast heart rate.

VALVULAR INSUFFICIENCY
Defective valves that close improperly, permitting a backflow of blood.

Vasoconstrictor
An impulse or agent that causes the muscles of the arterioles to constrict, raising blood pressure.

Vasodilator
An impulse or agent that causes the muscles of the arterioles to relax, lowering blood pressure.

Vein
Blood vessel that carries blood from various parts of the body back to the heart. All veins except the pulmonary veins carry unoxygenated blood. The pulmonary veins carry freshly oxygenated blood from the lungs to the heart.

Venous blood
Unoxygenated blood.

Ventricle
One of two pumping chambers of the heart. The left ventricle pumps oxygenated blood through the arteries to the body tissues, while the right ventricle pumps unoxygenated blood through the pulmonary artery to the lungs for reoxygenation.

Index